THE THYROID

PARADOX

How to Get the Best Care for Hypothyroidism

JAMES K. RONE, M.D.

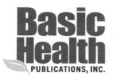

Basic Health
PUBLICATIONS, INC.

The information contained in this book is based upon the research and personal and professional experiences of the author. It is not intended as a substitute for consulting with your physician or other healthcare provider. Any attempt to diagnose and treat an illness should be done under the direction of a healthcare professional.

The publisher does not advocate the use of any particular healthcare protocol but believes the information in this book should be available to the public. The publisher and author are not responsible for any adverse effects or consequences resulting from the use of the suggestions, preparations, or procedures discussed in this book. Should the reader have any questions concerning the appropriateness of any procedures or preparation mentioned, the author and the publisher strongly suggest consulting a professional healthcare advisor.

Basic Health Publications, Inc.
28812 Top of the World Drive
Laguna Beach, CA 92651
949-715-7327 • www.basichealthpub.com

Library of Congress Cataloging-in-Publication Data
Rone, James K.
   The thyroid paradox : how to get the best care for hypothyroidism /
James K. Rone.
      p. cm.
   Includes bibliographical references and index.
   ISBN 978-1-59120-204-2
   1. Hypothyroidism. I. Title.

   RC657.R65   2007
   616.4'44—dc22

                                             2007003190

Editor: John Anderson
Typesetting/Book design: Gary A. Rosenberg
Cover design: Mike Stromberg

Printed in the United States of America

10   9   8   7   6   5   4   3   2   1

CONTENTS

ACKNOWLEDGMENTS

For inspiring this book, I thank my patients: they have been and are my greatest teachers. Many physicians and professors shaped me, through the facts and skills they taught or urged me to learn, and through their professionalism, which I continually strive to emulate. I cannot name them all, but a few (in no special order) are: Eugene Mayer, Abdul Ghaffar, Uwe Fohlmeister, Rob Perlstein, Bob Dons, Steve Breitzke, Kevin Tong, O'Neill Barrett, Paul Graham, Ed Quinones, and Charlie Reasner.

For editorial assistance, Meredith Wogan.

For life and commitment, my mother.

For all things, the late William E. Rone, Jr.—writer and father.

For love, support, and friendship always, Susan.

Paradox **1.** A seemingly contradictory statement that may nonetheless be true. **2.** One exhibiting inexplicable or contradictory aspects. **3.** An assertion that is essentially self-contradictory, though based on a valid deduction from acceptable premises. **4.** A statement contrary to received opinion.

—*American Heritage Dictionary of the English Language,*
4th edition

Hypothyroidism Diminished production of thyroid hormone, leading to thyroid insufficiency.

—*Illustrated Stedman's Medical Dictionary,*
24th edition

INTRODUCTION

Drawing from my personal and professional experience with hypo-thyroidism, *The Thyroid Paradox* scrutinizes a healthcare system tacking off course. The intended destination is the quality care of low-thyroid patients. The opposing forces? To quote Captain Reneau from the film *Casablanca*, "Round up the usual suspects." Suspects that include insurance carriers, government oversight and interference, and litigation run amok. These oft-blamed villains wreak as much havoc in the thyroid clinic as anywhere. But more egregious obstacles to identifying and treating hypothyroidism arise from within medicine itself, in the form of scientific stagnation and clinical simplism.

By scientific stagnation, I mean doctors thinking in overly dogmatic terms—the thyroid is this way, no other, and won't ever change. Among respected doctors at universities and research institutes who teach future and current doctors how to practice medicine, I see a pervasive resistance to entertaining any possibility that established thyroid doctrine might be, if not wrong, at least not entirely correct. Worse, I have witnessed a "conspiracy of silence" about the weaknesses of current thyroidology practice, despite supportive data published by that same academic elite.

The second half of the problem—clinical simplism—is embedded in the close-mindedness of the first half—and in the natural human tendency to follow paths of least resistance. If thyroid disease travels over a single metaphorical railroad track, then doctors in the trenches of real-world medicine need not waste much of their limited time per patient

1

wondering where a particular thyroid train is headed. Similarly, they needn't expend any imagination thinking beyond the obvious.

I allude here to honest but mistaken assumptions about the intricacies of thyroid disease. Some clinical simplism, though, is deliberate, imposed from outside the ranks of doctors, nurses, and other direct caregivers by institutions with agendas not necessarily devoted to your getting the most benefit out of your doctor-patient relationship.

HYPOTHYROIDISM IS UNDERDIAGNOSED

If you suffer from low thyroid, or think you might, and want to learn more—especially if you're dissatisfied with the answers you're getting from your doctor—this book is for you. We will not wallow in medico-socio-economic esoterica. The extent to which these matters occupy coming chapters will be offered only to postulate explanations for why modern health care in America so often, incongruously, does a lousy job—even fails, in some cases—at finding and fixing a relatively straightforward condition. What follows is an overview of thyroid physiology and the disorder resulting from thyroid hormone insufficiency—*hypothyroidism*. A condition known to be common that *paradoxically* may be rampantly overlooked.

How common is hypothyroidism? One summary of studies published between 1977 and 1995 indicates that almost 1 percent of women in the United States, Europe, and Japan suffers from hypothyroidism. Men too are affected, but less often. More recent research claims that 5.8 percent of females and 3.4 percent of males above the age of twelve in the United States are hypothyroid. Yet, hypothyroidism is underdiagnosed. Peer-reviewed research supports this fact. In my opinion, though, the problem is even worse than mainstream research indicates. The question is not whether we miss hypothyroidism, but rather how much of it do we miss?

Many people have complaints consistent with low thyroid (fatigue, for example), yet they have never been tagged with a thyroid diagnosis. Two possible reasons are that they don't have a thyroid problem, or they do and it's been overlooked. Perhaps their doctors never checked, never measured blood thyrotropin levels (which is how almost all hypothyroidism is found nowadays). Or perhaps they did blood work and declared it "normal." In any given case, of course, the doctor might be right. Fatigue, for example, has many dozens of possible causes, ranging from the normal physiologic response to overexertion to deadly malignancies. In fact, all chronic diseases are probably associated with some degree of fatigue. Sometimes, however, the thyroid system is defective in these people, but in a way too subtle or obscure to be easily detected. In other words, the doctor could be wrong.

Remember the 1 percent to 6 percent of women that research says are hypothyroid? That data came from studies labeling people low thyroid only when blood tests proved it. How accurate are those tests and do they miss anybody? I think they do. Low thyroid is common, everybody knows it's common, yet cases are missed.

That is the titular *paradox*.

MY EXPERIENCE AS BOTH PHYSICIAN AND PATIENT

Much information about hypothyroidism is at your fingertips via the Internet, libraries, bookstores, magazines, and word of mouth, not to mention your doctor. As a user of such resources, this book included, you owe it to yourself to be critical. Consider the source and make certain there is adequate reason to trust that source. If you're reading this, you're probably not a person with unquestioning faith in your doctor's opinion. If you're skeptical or just want to explore alternatives, I suggest you seek out several references so you don't wind up following anything too radical or dangerous. My wife won't buy a toaster without scouring *Consumer Reports*. At least as much caution is warranted when seeking health advice.

Why listen to me? I am a practicing physician, licensed in two states, and board certified in endocrinology—the subspecialty of internal medicine dealing with hormone disorders. The focus and passion of my practice since 1990 has been thyroid disease. I am a member of the American Thyroid Association and the Endocrine Society, and a Fellow of the American College of Endocrinology and the American College of Physicians. I have authored textbook chapters and published in national and international journals. And, I'm a low-thyroid patient myself. My diagnosis was based on mild blood-work irregularities that many doctors, even today, ignore. No doubt exists in my mind, however, that thyroid pills have benefited my health and well-being.

My experience as a patient has made me more sensitive as a doctor to the idea that mild or barely recognizable thyroid irregularities can be significant and worthy of treatment. My scientifically grounded colleagues might dismiss my personal stake in this story as "anecdotal" and unworthy of inclusion in a serious academic debate. That's a reasonable concern, which is why I cite published research throughout to bolster my arguments. My opinions may be biased, but the research backing them isn't.

Bottom line: I am uniquely qualified to write a book straddling the fences of low-thyroid opinion. I have a foot in three camps, that of: (1) thyroid patient, (2) mainstream endocrinologist, and (3) medical heretic concerned that low-thyroid patients are too often overlooked.

IRRECONCILABLE DIFFERENCES?

Navigating out of the thyroid paradox requires an understanding of the various approaches medical practitioners take in dealing with thyroid problems. You need to know where your doctor, author, herbalist, or tribal shaman is coming from before deciding whether to embrace his or her advice. Let's start with two fundamental dichotomies in the hypothyroidism debate: specialists versus generalists, and mainstreamists versus reformists.

Specialists versus Generalists

There are understandable differences between how an endocrinologist might manage a thyroid patient and how a family doctor might. The blunt truth is your physician may not know everything about thyroid disease. However, I could say the same about any doctor on any subject—twenty-first-century medicine is too vast to be mastered by any individual. I consider myself to be quite an authority on the thyroid, but would never recommend me as the physician to treat your sinus infection or do your gallbladder surgery. Yet, thyroid patients are often not referred to a specialist. One reason is primary-care providers (PCPs) tend to view thyroid disease as being pretty cut-and-dried. Often it is, and thyroid problems, however bad, are rarely life-threatening.

A cardiologist once told me, "When the thyroid fails, they don't call it 'the Big One'." True enough. Consequently, the typical PCP will be more comfortable with a thyroid issue—either handling it or ignoring it—than with, for example, an irregular heartbeat. Even when a PCP wants to refer, it can be easier said than done. In 1999, there were only 2,389 endocrinologists serving adults in office-based practice in the United States. This is an average of less than fifty per state and an estimated 12 percent fewer than needed.

When nonspecialists do wade into a suspected case of hypothyroidism, they tend to fall back on what they learned in medical school and residency. PCPs have been taught it's all about numbers, and anyone saying otherwise is a dangerous quack. If laboratory results are normal, the problem can't be the thyroid. I know, because I've drilled that dogma into the skulls of many students and residents myself. Some refer to this approach as the "tyranny of the test." Even an endocrinologist might arrive at the conclusion that "It's not your thyroid." And, of course, it might not be. However, after years of focusing on the thyroid—the Rodney Dangerfield ("I don't get no respect") of organs—controversies, chinks in the armor of traditional thyroidology, became apparent to me. If you're a low-thyroid patient being treated by your PCP, and everything seems fine, there's probably no reason to bother with a specialist. But if you're not feeling better—especially if you were told, "It's not your thyroid" and the investigation ended there—you should be aware that an endocrinology referral would be a reasonable next step. There are differences in knowledge, skill, and aggressiveness between specialists and generalists. Be warned, though: endocrinologists are as (or even more) responsible for creating and perpetuating the thyroid paradox as PCPs.

Mainstreamists versus Reformists

I sort physicians and others caring for and pontificating about thyroid disease into two groups: mainstreamists and reformists. Mainstreamists adhere to the typically accepted principles of modern Western medicine. Reformists, on the other hand, generally espouse that hypothyroidism is grossly underdiagnosed; that the usual tests and therapies are weak at best and useless at worst; and that thyroid pills fix pretty much everything, if you take a lot in just the right form and if you ignore pesky safety concerns. I don't consider either group to be entirely right or entirely wrong. About matters unproven, I think mainstreamists tend to be overly close-minded, and reformists tend to be overly open-minded.

Do I, a solidly mainstream physician, go along with thyroid reformists? I do, to a point. It is a poor scientist who refuses to question, to recognize that what is accepted could be wrong, or at least incomplete. An article in the British medical journal *Lancet* stated that there are "a few things we know, a few things we think we know (but probably don't), and lots of things we don't know."

Medicine bears a greater burden than other scientific fields. In it, both bad science and lack of good science affects lives. If a drug turns out to be dangerous, or a life-saving one takes too long to pass muster, people die. Physicians are therefore obligated to be more liberal thinkers than other scientists. They must see beyond pure data and become accustomed to operating in an environment where important facts remain unknown. A good doctor is neither paralyzed by, nor reckless in, such an informational void. It is a cliché, but medicine is both science and art.

Part of being a good doctor is balancing the art and the science of medical practice. Choices about testing and treatment are made based not only on science, but on cost, insurance coverage, and a range of patient-specific issues such as fear, indecision, cultural barriers, frustration, treatment side effects, misunderstandings, and outright irrational refusals. Juggling it all with compassion and efficacy is the physician's lot and a truly artistic endeavor. How does this relate to the thyroid paradox? Some of what I will propose, however reasonable I (and hopefully you) think it sounds, has not been validated by "science" as it is typically applied to medical decision-making today. But, as I said, good medicine is not all science.

Origins of What We Know or Think We Know

Mainstreamist opinions about thyroid disease stray little from the standards of care followed by most licensed physicians. Those standards draw from the experience of generations of doctors and from peer-reviewed research. *Peer-reviewed* means the information was published in a journal whose editorial board assured that the paper met their criteria for quality data collection and that it drew reasonable conclusions from those data. If so, it is "good data," likely to be accurate and deserving of an audience. This process is designed to ensure no "bad data" gets out (nothing that is wrong, inadequately substantiated, or plain dangerous), but that doesn't mean all good data sees the light of day. Editors reject papers for many reasons, ranging from lack of page space to the reputation of the author, or lack thereof. The process whereby knowledge is passed down to working doctors is rife with human bias, judgment, and error. The part of this process we tend to regard as pure science, therefore, is anything but. I'm not entirely critical of this process. When the prestigious *Journal of Clinical Endocrinology and Metabolism* reports something, it carries weight. Doctors the world over will believe it and run with it. The *Journal's* editorial board must therefore be cautious. Mistakes could do harm. Better to reject ten good studies than to let a bad one slip through.

Thus, mainstream thyroidology is rooted in two tar pit-like institutions: the "this is the way we've always done it and always will" phalanx and the hard-to-break-into world of peer-reviewed publishing. Very fertile ground, I'm afraid, for close-mindedness.

Reformists, on the other hand, make bold assertions about hypothyroidism that often haven't been tested to the satisfaction of conventional medicine. I didn't say reformist approaches are necessarily wrong, they just haven't been proven. The problem is that to the pure mainstreamist almost any degree of uncertainty is unpalatable. That's a hard line to take, but at stake is a person's health. If something unproven turns out to be worthless, that's bad enough, but what if the unproven course causes side effects that aggravate a patient's circumstances? These can be very complex issues and reformists too readily gloss over them. There are some legitimate therapies with very real benefits, for example, that also carry very serious risks. How do you balance risk versus benefit and make the right choice?

One of the basic doctrines of conventional Western medicine is *primum non nocere:* "first, do no harm." That means, physicians prefer to err on the side of doing nothing rather than risk making a patient worse. What if I can offer, though, a nonstandard treatment that I don't think will hurt, but in my gut I feel is likely to help? First, there's a considerable gulf between "I don't think it will hurt" and "It's almost certainly safe." For the sake of argument, though, let's assume this magic pill is 100 percent safe. Doesn't my patient deserve the benefit of the doubt—to be given the treatment—if it is safe and might help? Mainstreamists say "no," reformists say "yes," and I lean cautiously toward *yes.*

In statistics, you run across a thing called "*p* value." *P* stands for "probability"—the probability that some event, like a patient improving after taking a pill, happened solely by chance (in other words, the probability that the drug did nothing). It is universal in mainstream research to require a *p* value of less than (<) 0.05 for results to be called significant. That is, for a treatment to be accepted, a study must demonstrate not only that subjects were helped, but that there is at least a 95 percent chance the treatment did the helping, rather than some act of God or other factor. Sounds great.

Let's change the numbers, though. Say the same study still indicates that a greater portion felt better in the group that got treatment than the group that didn't, but this time there is only a 90 percent chance the treatment is responsible ($p < 0.10$). The resulting journal article will declare no statistically significant benefit and doctors the world over will reject the therapy. Or, if they do accept it, they will do so very marginally. "Come on!" I think—if there is no demonstrable harm (a big *if*, but we're being hypothetical here), and *if* the proportion of patients who benefited looks substantial to the naked eye—most patients would take the pill if told there was a 90 percent chance it was responsible for that substantial benefit. And I would tend to agree with them. Yet, published papers and clinical practice guidelines will insist the treatment is unproven and not recommended.

Reformist authors argue their treatments work because patients feel better. They are safe because they haven't seen bad outcomes. I for one can't recall witnessing a death from penicillin allergy, but it happens hundreds of times every year. My point is, just because something feels good doesn't necessarily mean it's safe and healthy. Reformist enthusiasm for their interventions is understandable, even commendable. Faced with a miserable patient, a physician wants to help. In some cases, though, this altruism drives innovative doctors to bypass the arduous steps—and glacial speed—of clinical research and peer-reviewed publication. It's hard for radical ideas to make it into a top journal, so the frustrated reformist goes directly to the patient. Who guarantees that intervention works and is safe? Peer-reviewed research offers a safety net in the mainstream world; reformists and their patients may be working without a net.

Open-mindedness is a two-way street. Mainstreamists should not so harshly condemn interventions that are logical but not proven beyond a reasonable doubt. Reformists must be cognizant of the possibility that these treatments might do harm, or at least might not help. Unfortunately, both reformists and mainstreamists, tend to be close-minded in their own ways.

Cookbook Medicine

Reformists' recommendations grow largely from observation, supposition, and individual experience. The medical establishment at the same time has been drifting further from defining "good care" based on these factors. A wedge is being driven between mainstreamists and reformists, forcing open a fissure in whatever common ground might have existed. This wedge goes by the name of evidence-based medicine (EBM), the current mantra in every hospital, clinic, medical school, and third-party payer's office. Dr. Victor Montori, an endocrinologist at the Mayo Clinic in Rochester, Minnesota, defines EBM as the "judicious use of the best available evidence from clinical research in making clinical decisions." This evidence then goes into creating so-called clinical practice guidelines, which are publications that define and publicize standards of care. Doctors these days are encouraged to seek scientific justification for everything done to and for patients. Reliance upon instinct and intellect is being bred out of the modern mainstream physician. "Cookbook medicine" has arrived.

Whether that's good or bad is the heart of the thyroid paradox. Should doctors rest on science and follow published standards blindly and throw out common sense? That's what mainstreamists are doing. The problem with unquestioned adherence to evidence-based medicine and clinical practice guidelines is that they are often incomplete, and sometimes wrong.

Until mid-2002, for example, hardly anyone questioned prescribing years of estrogen replacement to postmenopausal women. Then the Women's Health Initiative study stunned everyone by showing that women who took a certain estrogen product suffered more heart attacks and strokes than those who didn't. What had seemed an obvious good idea was suddenly found to be dangerous. The standard of care for postmenopausal women changed, literally overnight.

The estrogen story is relevant to our thyroid discussion. The first lesson we can learn from it is that we cannot assume we know all the long-term effects of loading up on hormones that have naturally ceased production. In other words, without good evidence that a certain low thyroid hormone level is truly abnormal *and* harmful, we must be circumspect about giving treatment. We shouldn't assume that taking a thyroid pill is safe just because our bodies make the stuff naturally and it makes us feel better. Until more study is done on thyroid pills given in nonstandard situations, we must fall back on a concept foreign to the evidence-based doctor—common sense. And, from that perspective, if thyroid hormone makes people feel better and it seems safe, why not use it?

Lesson two from the estrogen debacle: Be extremely cautious about treatments yet to be subjected to rigorous testing for safety and effectiveness, no matter how good they sound. It's easy to become scientifically lazy, to trust our eyes and ears and logic and charge forth into therapeutic folly. I'm not saying don't take thyroid hormone or that we shouldn't be giving it more frequently. I am saying thyroid hormone is a potent prescription drug that demands respect for the good and the bad it can do.

There's a time and place for a good doctor to rely on his or her gut, and a time and place to follow the cookbook. It's when we try to go completely one way or the other that we get into trouble. The mathematician Alfred North Whitehead said, "There are no whole truths; all truths are half truths. It is trying to treat them as whole truths that plays the devil." Too often mainstreamists and reformists draw lines in the sand neither will cross, even if it seems reasonable to do so.

I agree with reformists that current thyroid testing has weaknesses and that hypothyroidism is underdiagnosed. I have felt conflicted over the disconnect between my reformist instincts and my mainstreamist training. Even different phases of my training conflicted. In medical school and residency, my sage guides counseled: "Treat the patient, not the numbers." Yet, endocrinologists are taught the opposite: "Treat the numbers, not the patient."

Is there a happy medium? Reformists risk a lot by disposing of the scientific method. Yet, those strictly adhering to science and Hippocratic ("first, do no harm") doctrine are obliged to recognize gaps in our knowledge, work to fill those gaps, and in the interim be a little flexible, and humble. Doctors on the front lines, meanwhile, must be cautious but proactive, using every available tool when evaluating the patient who may be low thyroid. Thyroid testing should be interpreted, not in a vacuum, but as part of a diagnostic process based on the preponderance of evidence, not any single kernel of it. Treatment, when it seems reasonable, should be undertaken using U.S. Food and Drug Administration–approved products, dispensed according to a licensed practitioner's prescription and supervision.

AN OPEN-MINDED APPROACH

The Thyroid Paradox is for the person who's been told, "It's not your thyroid," without then being told, convincingly, what it *is* if it's not your thyroid. Maybe you've been told nothing is wrong and know darn well something is. There must be some reason, some fix, for that chronic fatigue, body aching, weight gain, dry skin, constipation, "brain fog," depression, and menstrual irregularity. Your answer might or might not be found in these pages, but if low thyroid levels are involved, chances are you will find help here.

This little book, by the way, is not a guide to everything about the thyroid. Some publications try to do that and, if interested in a broader view, you should seek them out to augment my coverage. Largely untouched in this volume are important disorders like hyperthyroidism (high thyroid), thyroid nodules, and thyroid cancer. We will *only* be examining hypothyroidism. For an authoritative and comprehensive mainstream thyroid manual, I suggest *Your Thyroid: A Home Reference* by Lawrence Wood, M.D., David Cooper, M.D., and Chester Ridgway, M.D. (4th ed., Ballantine Books, 2005); or *Overcoming Thyroid Problems* by Jeffrey Garber, M.D. (McGraw-Hill, 2005)—world-class thyroidologists all. For something a bit more "alternative," *The Thyroid Solution* by Ridha Arem, M.D., (Ballantine Books, 2000) has a lot to recommend it.

The primary goal of *The Thyroid Paradox* is to correct the pervasive oversimplification of thyroid science and of most of the care given to thyroid patients today. In the common view of how the thyroid system works, the brain talks to the pituitary, then the pituitary talks to the thyroid, and the thyroid begets its hormone, which ventures forth to do all sorts of good stuff all over the body. That view is correct, as far as it goes. Today's doctors have good tests—as far as *they* go—to evaluate this brain-pituitary-thyroid-body circuit. Unfortunately, an overtrusting, shortsighted approach to interpreting those tests can lead well-meaning physicians to miss problems. The opinion held by most physicians, including top people in the field, is that the majority of low-thyroid cases are caused by a dysfunctional thyroid gland. No short circuit in the brain, no loose bolt in the pituitary, nothing in the zillion downstream physiochemical events that have to happen for thyroid hormone to work. Rule Number One: the thyroid gland is the only place anything ever goes wrong.

Does that make sense? It doesn't to me and, to be frank, I too am guilty of oversimplifying here. Nobody claims that Rule Number One is never broken. Pituitary problems, for example, are well known to disrupt thyroid function. But such exceptions are almost universally said to be rare. What if they aren't? That is the thrust of this book—in thyroid disease, exceptions may be as much or more common than the rule.

The simple (and cheap) approach to hypothyroidism is to follow the crowd, to never think beyond what's taught in medical schools. Namely, if there is no evident problem in the thyroid gland proper, then hypothyroidism is virtually ruled out. Even if that statement accurately reflected reality—and I don't think it does—the *virtually* part is routinely forgotten. The complex approach to hypothyroidism, on the other hand, is to be open-minded about possible exceptions to Rule Number One, to think outside the box.

The Thyroid Paradox explores when to consider drifting beyond the bounds of thyroidological doctrine, and how far it might be safe to do so. Nothing here should be construed as advice to self-diagnose or self-treat. You should never change your dose of thyroid medicine without checking with your prescribing physician or at least seeking the face-to-face opinion of another qualified doctor. This book is meant to enhance office visits, to spark questions and discussion. It might convince you to seek a second opinion or subspecialty referral. I hope, above all, that it helps.

CHAPTER 1

THYROID BOOT CAMP

This chapter lays out the thyroid knowledge base necessary to understand the science and terms used throughout this book. A glossary is also provided at the end of the book to clarify technical terms as they arise.

THYROID ANATOMY AND PHYSIOLOGY

The thyroid gland is a roughly U-shaped organ at the front of the neck beneath the Adam's apple. (Some people refer to their "thyroids," but each of us has only one.) The gland has two lobes about two inches tall each, which rest vertically alongside the voice box and windpipe. The normal weight of an adult's thyroid is about 20 grams (0.7 ounces).

Though small, the thyroid is the human body's largest pure endocrine gland. A gland is any structure that secretes something within or outside the body. Glands can be endocrine or exocrine. Examples of exocrine glands include the liver, most of the pancreas, sweat and salivary glands, and the breasts. These organs secrete products by way of tubes called ducts onto the skin or into a body cavity, never into blood. Endocrine glands, on the other hand, secrete substances called hormones directly into the bloodstream. From head to foot, the major endocrine glands are the pituitary, the thyroid, the parathyroids, the adrenals, the pancreatic islet cells, and the gonads (testes in men, ovaries in women).

Hormones are substances produced in one part of the body that travel to another part via the bloodstream in order to exert some kind of control. In partnership with the nervous system, hormones are the body's means of communicating with itself. Nerve signals are electrical and rapid; hormonal ones are slow, but last longer, and are chemical in nature.

Some hormones are small proteins (for example, insulin and growth hormone) or sugar-protein hybrids (thyrotropin). These bind to a receptor on a cell's surface, triggering a series of actions inside—like a biological Rube Goldberg device. Other hormones penetrate cells and interact directly with DNA; go straight to the top, so to speak. Steroid hormones (like estrogen, testosterone, and cortisol) work this way. Thyroid hormone is unique. It is essentially a tiny protein that works like a steroid. It walks right up to DNA and barks out its orders, perhaps an underappreciated clue to the thyroid system's importance.

A normal thyroid gland often can't be felt. An enlarged one is called a goiter. In addition to suffering more thyroid disease than men, women often have bigger thyroids, a fact that resulted in some humorous historical misconceptions. The thyroid was discovered by the Greek physician Galen, who treated mauled gladiators in the second century A.D., but it took until the late 1800s for scientists to determine the organ's function. Along the way came much wild speculation. During the 1600s, for example, someone declared the thyroid existed simply to fill out and beautify the neck, which, naturally, was why women had bigger ones.

Structurally, the thyroid consists of microscopic spheres called follicles, each of which is a self-contained hormone factory. A thyroid follicle is like a piece of chocolate candy with a caramel center. Like the chocolate, follicular cells form an outer shell; a substance called colloid lies at the center like the filling. Colloid looks like bubble gum under a microscope and is composed of thyroglobulin, a large protein produced by follicular cells and secreted inward, toward the core of the sphere. Thyroid hormone is manufactured and stored within thyroglobulin. The thyroid actually warehouses a huge amount of its namesake product, enough to meet the body's needs for months. No other endocrine gland does this— another testament, perhaps, to a critical role for thyroid hormone in proper body functioning.

How important is the thyroid? We've already mentioned three clues suggesting it is tremendously important: (1) the thyroid is the largest pure endocrine gland, (2) its hormone acts directly on DNA, and (3) large amounts of it are stored. Here are an additional three: (1) a thyroid gland is found in every vertebrate species, from fish to lizards to mammals, (2) it is the first endocrine organ to form in the human embryo, starting a mere twenty-four days after conception, and finally, (3) in adults, the thyroid receives, gram for gram, 50 percent more blood flow than the kidneys.

THYROID HORMONES

The dietary nutrient iodine is needed to make thyroid hormone. Follicular cells trap it from the blood, making the thyroid, in effect, a powerful iodine sponge. Iodine molecules then get hooked onto thyroglobulin. Like all proteins, thyroglobulin is made up of amino acid building blocks. One of the twenty common amino acids in humans is tyrosine. It is onto the tyrosines within thyroglobulin that iodine becomes chemically bonded. Then, a pair of iodine-enriched tyrosines couple like railroad cars to form a unit called an iodothyronine.

When the body needs thyroid hormone, follicular cells bite off and swallow pieces of colloid (composed of thyroglobulin). Iodothyronines are pruned off and get spit out the other end of the follicular cell, toward the outside of the sphere, into the bloodstream. If a bud containing three iodines is snipped, the resulting hormone is called triiodothyronine (T_3). Clippings containing four iodines form thyroxine (T_4), the most abundant product of the thyroid gland.

Thyroxine (T_4) is the major circulating thyroid hormone, although half of each day's output is converted to triiodothyronine (T_3) by removing one of the four iodines. Much of this postproduction work happens in the liver and kidneys. Other important sites include the brain, pituitary, and skeletal muscle. Conversion of T_4 into T_3 is key to proper thyroid system function because T_3 is the more powerful hormone—at least three times more potent than T_4. In fact, most of us consider T_4 to be a pro-hormone, an immature substance that must be switched on (via transformation to T_3). T_4 originates only in the thyroid gland, while T_3 is issued both from the thyroid and from this peripheral conversion occurring throughout the body.

There are also minor thyroid hormones. Examples include T_1 and T_2 (containing one or two iodines, respectively), reverse T_3 (in which the three iodines are shuffled differently), and various conjugated thyroid hormones (in which extra molecules get tacked on, generally rendering the hormone more vulnerable to destruction). Most of these minor forms seem to have some biologic activity—that is, they in some way mimic the actions of thyroid hormone, often at a weaker level than T_4 or T_3. Researchers are uncertain whether these effects are of any importance. What is certain is that doctors virtually never pay them any attention. (Some drug companies are starting to, however, and we may soon see "designer" thyroid hormone products appearing on pharmacists' shelves.)

WHY IS THE THYROID IMPORTANT?

Why do we have thyroid hormone? Thyroid hormone increases the body's metabolic rate, that is, sets your engine's idle speed. We're talking about the metabolic rate of every system, every organ, and every tissue in the human body. That covers a lot of ground. One of the most important thyroid effects in warm-blooded animals is thermogenesis, the generation of body heat. Each calorie we eat has three possible fates: it can be stored (as glycogen, fat, or protein), converted into energy for work, or burned to produce body heat. Thyroid hormone is one of the traffic cops directing calories down one pathway or another.

Thyroid hormone increases oxygen consumption, body temperature, and protein synthesis. It degrades fat and enhances both absorption and the processing of carbohydrates. Thyroid hormone accelerates pulse rate and strengthens the pumping force of the heart; it dilates blood vessels, and increases the volume per minute of blood circulated through the body. Brain activity is stimulated, as is muscle vigor. Thyroid hormone promotes the production of many substances, including enzymes that regulate chemical reactions—speeding up, among other things, removal of drugs and toxins from the body. Most of these effects occur ploddingly by way of the interaction of T_3 with DNA. But other effects, including many cardiovascular ones, are direct and immediate.

The cardiologist's joke about thyroid failure not being "the Big One" recognizes the obvious: a sick heart is usually more devastating than a sick thyroid. That fact, however, does not mean we should dismiss the critical role played by the thyroid system. The implications of slowed metabolism in tissues all over the body are huge, if insidious. A few days, weeks, or even months of low thyroid may be of little lasting consequence. But years of it, untreated or inadequately treated, could be catastrophic, hobbling the function of every organ.

Under these circumstances, for example, the heart doesn't pump oxygen-carrying blood as strongly, even to its own coronary arteries, possibly leading to angina (chest pain caused by poor oxygen delivery to the heart muscle). Blood pressure and cholesterol levels elevate, creating an increased risk of heart attack and stroke. Brain function diminishes, leading to poor concentration and loss of efficiency at work or school, affecting promotions and grades. Depression may ensue, interfering with relationships and resulting in suicidal thoughts and actions. Drugs may be prescribed over the years for hypertension, cholesterol, and depression, inflicting their own side effects and costs. Clearly, a properly functioning thyroid system is vital to your overall health.

CONTROL OF THE THYROID SYSTEM

There are two major levels of thyroid system control—analogous to coarse and fine tuning on an old television set:

- Regulation of production and secretion of thyroid hormone from the thyroid gland

- Regulation of T_4 to T_3 peripheral conversion

The first of these, production and secretion of thyroid hormone, is overseen by the pituitary gland—what our health teachers called the "master gland." Located beneath the brain and behind the eyes, the pituitary is attached to and takes orders from the hypothalamus, a part of the brain that regulates circadian rhythms, body temperature, heart rate, water retention, sweating, appetite and thirst, and basic behaviors and reactions such as anger, fear, horror, and sexual aggression. When thyroid hormone is deemed lacking, the hypothalamus secretes thyrotropin-releasing hormone (TRH), which descends along nerves to the pituitary, where it stimulates production and secretion of thyrotropin, also known as thyroid-stimulating hormone (TSH). TSH enters the bloodstream and circulates to the thyroid gland, where it binds to receptors on follicular cells and orders the synthesis and release of thyroid hormone.

Just as your home furnace switches off when the room's temperature rises to match the thermostat setting, release of TSH ceases when thyroid hormone levels reach the set point established by the hypothalamus. Thus, a yin-yang relationship exists between thyroid hormone and TSH. As thyroid hormone levels fall, TSH rises to halt the decline. As thyroid hormone rises, TSH falls to prevent overactivation of the thyroid gland (hyperthyroidism). This part of the thyroid system, whereby the brain and pituitary regulate the thyroid gland, is called the hypothalamic-pituitary-thyroid (HPT) axis.

The second level of control, the fine-tuning, occurs in target organs that use and respond to thyroid hormone. Most tissues contain some version of an enzyme called deiodinase. Deiodinases activate or deactivate T_4 depending on local needs. Liver and kidney deiodinases manufacture, via T_4 to T_3 conversion, most of the T_3 found in the blood. Other organs, such as the brain, have their own deiodinases to tailor thyroid levels to their unique requirements.

Stable T_3 levels are vital to one's well-being, keeping each cell's metabolism tuned up and well oiled. If Nancy's liver were to detect a plunge in blood T_4, would that trigger a decrease in T_3 production, making Nancy feel suddenly exhausted? No, because deiodinases kick in. They convert a greater portion of available T_4 into T_3, therefore Nancy's T_3 levels never fall and she feels fine—in the short run.

But what if her thyroid gland had been surgically removed a month ago and she'd neglected to get filled the thyroid hormone prescription written by her doctor? By now, her T_4 is very low. Her body's only source of T_4 was her now-absent thyroid gland. For the first few weeks, her deiodinases manufacture enough T_3 to keep her metabolic engine running. But there is one organ that absolutely must have T_4: the brain. Proper thyroid levels are so critical to brain function that the brain excludes T_3 from external sources in the body and makes its own out of T_4 using a special deiodinase. At some point, then, when Nancy's T_4 levels drop low enough, liver and other peripheral conversion halts. What little T_4 remains is reserved for her brain.

So, depending on many factors, weighing the needs of an individual tissue versus those of the whole person, more or less T_3 gets made from T_4. This is the thyroid version of precision tuning. Unfortunately, deiodinase action is a black box, hidden from us inside millions of individual cells. Here lies a big problem with current thyroid testing. Most measurements of thyroid activity focus on that first, coarse level of control—the HPT axis. We can check T_3 levels, but only what's in the blood. What's going on within tissues, within cells—whether deiodinase is doing its job—can only be inferred from indirect evidence.

A possible third control mechanism—not generally recognized—lies between the HPT axis and peripheral conversion. This process involves serum transport proteins, little freight cars that haul thyroid hormone around in the blood. Even among endocrinologists, this part of the system receives very little attention, beyond the fact it interferes with certain blood tests, yet the impact of these proteins is staggering. Of all the T_4 in the bloodstream at any one time, more than 99 percent is glommed onto by transport proteins. This bound hormone is sequestered, prevented from doing anything useful, or so says conventional thyroidology.

Why make something as important as thyroid hormone, then waste almost all of it? The most logical explanation is that it is not wasted. Serum transport proteins probably represent a second storehouse of available hormone—waiting out in the hinterlands of the body to be released when and where needed. Later, we'll introduce a more intriguing possibility—that transport proteins are responsible for the deliberate and precise delivery of T_4 to individual cells.

Additional influences on thyroid function are incompletely understood and include psychological stress, starvation, severe illness, and numerous drugs.

Therefore, thyroid hormone levels are regulated or otherwise altered four different ways. To recap:

- The hypothalamic-pituitary-thyroid (HPT) axis
- Peripheral conversion of T_4 into T_3
- Serum transport proteins
- Interference from "wild card" factors (stress, starvation, illness, drugs)

However, only the HPT axis is routinely tested. Might doctors miss something when confidently declaring patients' thyroid tests normal? What about deiodinase problems or transport protein problems? Or subtle defects in the HPT axis, especially in the hypothalamic-pituitary part? Not only is it possible that things are being missed, I find it *impossible* to believe that they're not.

CHAPTER 2

WHEN TO THINK
LOW THYROID

At an office Christmas party, I groused to a senior internist my frustration over the inability of our veterinarian to provide a clear laboratory diagnosis of my cat's suspected hypothyroidism. I compared the dismal state of modern feline thyroid testing to the similar, if less profound, inadequacy of testing in humans. My elder chuckled, sagely replying, "You think it's bad *now*." He proceeded to tell me of the bad old days when the diagnosis of hypothyroidism was largely *clinical*—a physician's way of saying, "seat of the pants." They relied on the patient's story and a hands-on examination. He described hours obsessing over slowed reflexes, but he couldn't remember the name of the device for measuring them. I couldn't help, because I'd never done such a thing. By the time I trained, we were confident in our ability to diagnose all cases of low thyroid via laboratory tests. I learned the signs and symptoms to look for, but biochemistry trumped clinical evaluation every time.

The pendulum has swung the other way. My colleague lamented the lack of biochemical tools in his early days, but now we are dangerously close to throwing away his bedside clinical skills. ("Clinical" refers to a doctor's eyes, ears, hands, and head—what he or she does at the bedside. "Biochemical" is what the lab does, the application of technology.) Today's patients are no doubt better off. In the past, low thyroid was sometimes missed until the patient slipped into myxedema coma, the often-fatal result of years of untreated thyroid failure. I, however, have never seen true myxedema coma because improvements in technology and our reliance upon it have kept us from missing severe disease. What we *are* missing is mild low thyroid, a preferable but nevertheless suboptimal state of affairs.

It is not laziness that leads to glossing over history taking and examination. There may be some of that, but many doctors simply don't have time—too many patients, too few hours. One answer, of course, is to spend more time with each patient, but the realities of modern health care make that difficult. HMOs, institutional systems, and some large private offices may have quotas for doctors to meet. Even physicians in regular private practice feel pressure. With insurance payouts down and office overhead up—including crisis malpractice premiums and salaries for staff to satisfy onerous government regulations—more patients can mean the difference between making ends meet or not. All this as medical knowledge and technology expand—more stuff to do and less time to do it in. Given that, the lowly thyroid gets elbowed aside or at least left for a blood test to cover. Still, even physicians who do a good clinical assessment of the thyroid—and I know many—might be prematurely dissuaded from their suspicions by tests that may or may not reflect the patient's true status.

THE ZULEWSKI LIST

A 1997 paper by Zulewski and colleagues published in the *Journal of Clinical Endocrinology and Metabolism* correlated signs and symptoms with thyroid blood testing in 332 women. The authors defined "true" hypothyroidism using laboratory tests, but they discussed tissue hypothyroidism as something distinct from biochemical hypothyroidism, acknowledging a potential disconnect between thyroid hormone blood levels and what happens deep inside tissues and cells.

Besides providing a convenient list of low-thyroid findings, this article supports the critical need for history taking and exam. While concluding that routine blood tests are the best way to find patients with thyroid failure, the authors felt that signs and symptoms could be superior to blood work in determining severity of disease and in monitoring treatment. Of note, some subjects had high clinical scores (lots of signs and symptoms) but mild test abnormalities, supporting the notion that tissue thyroid deficiency can exist apart from obvious biochemical deficiency. Lab tests might not tell all.

The following is the Zulewski paper's list of clinical findings useful in identifying low-thyroid patients. The percentages show how often each symptom was found in people known to be hypothyroid.

- Delayed reflexes (77%)

- Dry skin (76%)

- Rough skin (60%)

- Puffiness (60%)

- Poor sweating (54%)

- Weight gain (54%)

- Tingling or burning (52%)

- Skin cold to the touch (50%)

- Constipation (48%)

- Slow movements (36%)

- Hoarseness (34%)

- Hearing loss (22%)

A score was calculated for each subject in the study, awarding one point for each of the symptoms found. People with a score of six or higher (that is, they had six or more of the twelve listed problems) were dubbed *clinically hypothyroid*. Those with two or fewer were labeled *normal*, and those in between were deemed *intermediate*.

The percentages beside each symptom in the list represent the sensitivity of that finding for identifying hypothyroidism. *Sensitivity* means positivity in disease. Mathematically, sensitivity is the percentage of all people with the disease in question (in this case hypothyroidism) who have a positive (that is, abnormal) test result. Here the search for symptoms and abnormal exam findings is considered a "test," just like a blood test. In the

Zulewski paper, delayed reflex was the most sensitive indicator of low thyroid, hearing loss the least.

Specificity is an equally important parameter when assessing the worth of any medical test. *Specificity* is negativity in the absence of disease. Mathematically, specificity is the percentage of all people without the disease who have a negative (that is, normal) result. A certain test (or finding) can be specific—hardly ever positive (present) except when the patient has the disease—without being sensitive, and vice versa.

Let me illustrate. Say a fisherman wants to catch tuna: he wants only tuna and wants to nab every single tuna in a certain square of ocean. If he drags a huge net behind his boat long enough, he might get every tuna, but he'll also get mackerel, grouper, barracuda, sharks, turtles, some seaweed, the odd World War II mine, and an old tire. The net is sensitive for tuna but not specific. So, our picky fisherman uses a pole instead, baited so only tuna will bite. But unless he cruises that square of ocean for a hundred years, I doubt he'll catch all the tuna. The pole is specific for tuna, but not sensitive.

What does any of this have to do with thyroidology? We want to catch all cases of hypothyroidism. The various tests at our disposal—history, examination, blood tests—are like the fisherman's nets and poles. Alone, none are ideal: any one test might miss a patient or tag one as low thyroid that isn't.

Though varying in sensitivity, the twelve items on the Zulewski list are pretty specific. None were found in more than 20 percent of normal people. Which means that any one of them might be found in up to 20 percent of normal people (whose thyroid systems work perfectly). Hence, the danger of relying on any single finding or test. Hoarseness might be caused by low thyroid or acute laryngitis or throat cancer. But if hoarseness coexists with several other problems on this list, hypothyroidism becomes a more likely explanation.

The following is a breakdown of clinical scores in the Zulewski paper—how many items were found out of the twelve—sorted by degree of known biochemical thyroid deficiency:

More serious thyroid deficiency (based on laboratory tests):

- 62% had clinical scores defining them as clinically hypothyroid.
- Most of the rest had intermediate scores.
- A few were clinically normal.

Less serious thyroid deficiency:

- 24% were clinically hypothyroid.
- About half had an intermediate score.
- About a quarter were normal.

This makes sense. The worse the laboratory abnormality, the more clinical features of hypothyroidism were found. But these patients are not our concern. Symptoms or no symptoms, they were already diagnosed with biochemical hypothyroidism and hadn't fallen through the cracks. Let's look instead at the 189 supposedly normal control subjects among the 332 women studied. All, according to the authors, had completely normal thyroid blood tests. If hypothyroidism is grossly underdiagnosed, as we've speculated, then a few of these normal people should have clinical hypothyroidism despite normal lab tests.

It turns out that almost 40 percent (according to my own analysis of data presented in the paper) of the control subjects had intermediate clinical scores. Four out of ten people meeting the researchers' definition of lab normalcy had three to five of the items on the list of common hypothyroid findings. A few had even more. Does that mean all 40 percent were hypothyroid? No, because the signs or symptoms might have been caused by something else. But it stands to reason that some were hypothyroid despite normal tests. The trick is figuring out which people with normal thyroid tests are actually deficient in thyroid hormone

FATIGUE

The Zulewski list is incomplete. For one thing, fatigue isn't on it. Nevertheless, most practitioners, including the authors of the American Association of Clinical Endocrinologists' clinical practice guidelines on thyroid disease, consider fatigue to be a cardinal feature of hypothyroidism. It was omitted from the Zulewski study probably because so many other things besides low thyroid can cause fatigue, including overexertion, psychiatric disease, and physical disorders of all kinds. In other words, while unremitting chronic fatigue may suggest something is amiss, it is worthless for narrowing down what that something is.

Fatigue is *nonspecific*. Most findings associated with low thyroid are and that's part of why biochemical testing is more respected than clinical evaluation in this field. Clinical evaluation is too nonspecific, but laboratory tests, I fear, may be too *nonsensitive*. That is, symptoms and signs (like fatigue) label people low thyroid who aren't and tests fail to label people low thyroid who are.

Returning to the fishing analogy, clinical assessment is like dragging a net—we catch all the tuna but snare a lot of other stuff too. Thyroid blood tests are like fishing poles—they hook only tuna, but a lot of tuna gets away. Neither tool by itself gets the job done, but if we use the net to gather all the tuna into one area, then throw our hook in the water, we might be getting somewhere. History, examination, and lab tests go hand in hand. We don't have the luxury of throwing any of them away.

WEIGHT GAIN

Body weight holds a special, cursed place in the thyroidologist's heart. Weight gain, or the inability to lose weight, are common complaints among the hypothyroid, or those convinced they are. Weight problems do appear on the Zulewski list and on that of most experts. Thyroidologists are quick to add, however, that the weight gain of hypothyroidism is mild and much of it is water; severe obesity due to low thyroid alone rarely, if ever, occurs.

Obesity, like fatigue, is nonspecific for hypothyroidism. It is also epidemic, its prevalence vastly exceeding the most generous estimates of thyroid disease frequency. Obesity has many roots, chief among them overeating and underexercising. Insulin resistance, the metabolic disorder underlying most diabetes, is also a frequent contributor.

Could low thyroid be a cause of obesity? In my opinion, absolutely; to think otherwise defies common sense. Low-thyroid patients are tired, tired people don't exercise, and lack of exercise leads to obesity. It's also logical that the lower metabolic rate and reduced thermogenesis (body heat production) of hypothyroidism would result in fewer calories being burned, thus increasing fat storage of those calories. I don't understand why this is so commonly denied. Such findings have been demonstrated, even reported in textbooks. One paper in the *Journal of Clinical Endocrinology and Metabolism* showed resting energy expenditure (calories burned per day when doing nothing) dropped by 15 percent when thyroid levels changed from borderline high to mildly low. More recently, a paper in the same periodical reported data on 4,082 Danes. Those who had a TSH between 2.0 and 3.6 milliunits per liter (mU/L)—the higher the TSH, the lower the thyroid hormone level—were 20 percent more likely to be obese than people with a TSH of 1.00–1.99 mU/L. And Danes with a TSH greater than 3.6 mU/L had twice the risk of obesity.

Yet the party line remains that obesity due to low thyroid doesn't happen. And to be fair, the Danish study could be used to support both points of view. Yes, people with a higher TSH piled on more pounds to a statistically significant degree, but over five years, not over six months. So, we're not looking at rapid weight gain. Also, regardless of TSH level, everybody in the study gained weight. Those with a higher TSH gained more, but there was no TSH level that prevented weight gain. And the average weight difference between the worst group and the best group was only about nine pounds.

So, thyroid hormone does affect weight, but it's probably not the sole reason somebody weighs three hundred pounds and can't lose it. Even under the best circumstances, losing weight and keeping it off are difficult. Disciplined lifestyle changes are mandatory. Our world seems dominated by two quests: (1) ever less need for physical exertion and (2) lots of tasty, convenient calories. That's why 120 million Americans (65 percent of the adult population) are overweight or frankly obese. Thyroid disease might contribute, but it's a small part of the problem.

Yet, patients bombard doctors every day with bitter complaints about weight and insist there must be a reason, like thyroid disease. To them, I say it would be a public health mistake for conscientious doctors to foster the myth that there is any reliable way to achieve and maintain weight loss without diet and exercise. And to claim any pill alone—thyroid hormone or any of the anti-obesity drugs—can permanently and safely solve a person's weight and fitness problems would almost always be a lie, or at least a false hope.

For example, say Diana gained one hundred pounds in two years and let's assume every last pound was because she was hypothyroid. Her eating and exercising stayed constant, but her body just didn't consume calories the way it should have. She gets diagnosed and put on a thyroid pill. Her thyroid levels normalize, and Diana's body is burning calories like a furnace again. She eats and exercises just as she did when she was a perfect size six. Does she lose the one hundred pounds?

Probably not. You see, if her energy intake and output are matching perfectly again, she won't gain more, but she won't lose either. To lose, she has to burn off about five hundred calories per day more than she takes in—through exercise and diet—until the one hundred pounds are gone. And this scenario assumes that every ounce of weight gain was due to thyroid disease, which is probably never true.

What if we give her a higher thyroid dose to boost her metabolism *above* normal, just long enough to get that one hundred pounds off? No pesky diet or exercise needed—problem solved? Nope. You're talking about making Diana hyperthyroid, which can cause a number of uncomfortable symptoms, not to mention serious problems like irregular heart rhythms, congestive heart failure, and stroke. Plus, the weight lost with hyperthyroidism is mostly muscle, not fat, resulting in weakness. It's not unheard of for people to use thyroid pills to take off pounds—it was a common practice until the 1980s—but any doctor today who deliberately causes hyperthyroidism as a weight-loss measure is, pure and simple, committing malpractice.

Whatever role the thyroid plays in a given person's obesity, treating an existing low-thyroid state should at least remove a stumbling block from the tortuous path of weight loss. Certainly people who have unusual difficulty losing weight, despite calorie reduction and exercise, deserve an open-minded evaluation of their thyroid function. Can low thyroid contribute to weight gain? Probably. Is thyroid treatment ever the sole fix? Unlikely.

OTHER CLUES TO HYPOTHYROIDISM

Additional signs and symptoms of low thyroid that didn't make the Zulewski list include the following:

- Drowsiness, poor memory, poor concentration

- Insomnia, irritability, anxiety

- Weakness, muscle cramps, joint pain, carpal tunnel syndrome

- Nausea, constipation

- Loss of interest in sex, infertility, menstrual problems

- Impotence

- Hair loss, brittle nails

- Mild blood pressure elevation

- Pale or yellowed skin

- Leakage of milk from the nipples

The presence of certain diseases may also signal the presence of a thyroid problem. For example, several serious nonthyroid conditions can arise out of the ashes of chronic thyroid deficiency. These include dyslipidemia (cholesterol/triglyceride problems), depression, heart attack, and a form of psychosis called myxedema madness. Also, a couple dozen or more diseases tend to show up in the same people as low thyroid, despite there being no cause-and-effect relationship. These include celiac sprue, type 1 diabetes, multiple sclerosis, lupus, rheumatoid arthritis, and sarcoidosis. In most cases, the link between these disorders and hypothyroidism is an inborn tendency toward autoimmunity, in which an overactive immune system turns on its owner like a rabid dog. People with one autoimmune disease often have others, and most thyroid problems are autoimmune in nature.

In summary, clinical alerts to a possible low-thyroid state include a long list of nonspecific signs and symptoms, fatigue and weight gain among them, and/or the presence of one or more diseases known to be caused by, or travel along with, hypothyroidism.

WHO NEEDS THYROID TESTING?

We've said hypothyroidism is common, so shouldn't everybody be tested? Drawing thyroid tests on everybody would be expensive and a waste of time and money for all who turn out to be healthy. That's not selfish, just practical. Also, there's a little thing called Bayes' theorem of conditional probability learned by every medical student. Bayes' theorem states that the more common a disease is in a group being tested, the more accurate the test. If I test every man, woman, and child in Kansas for Rare-as-Hen's-Teeth disease, even those with positive results probably aren't sick. They are more likely to be "false positives" than true positives. But if I only test those with symptoms of the disease, a positive result carries more weight. With testing, we want to stack the deck in favor of finding what-ever we're looking for. This is called increasing the pretest probability of disease.

Postmenopausal women are a group for which blanket thyroid testing has been advocated, because this group suffers a lot of thyroid disease. The pretest probability of disease in older women is high. Among those with a positive test result, more will be true positives than false positives, and the number of people who have to be tested to find one case of low thyroid falls into a reasonable range.

Something should be obvious from the above discussion, something to think about before insisting your doctor run any test he or she isn't keen on. Medical laboratory test results are sometimes wrong. In fact, they are so often wrong, doctors have a slang name for erroneous results: *labomas*. The reasons for labomas range from human error to unavoidable statisti-cal uncertainty to odd-ball antibodies mucking up the works on a molecu-lar level. I recall a medical school lecture in which the professor claimed that one in every twenty lab test results was wrong. That's why doctors usually repeat abnormal tests before doing anything about them.

The point is, testing for the heck of it is a bad idea. That said, there is interest in the generalized screening of adults for hypothyroidism. Screening means a fishing expedition—testing done in the absence of signs or symptoms of the disease in question. Like a healthy woman getting an annual Pap smear or mammogram. Hypothyroidism does meet the usual criteria justifying screening: it's an important common disease (worth finding), easily treated (we can do something about it if we find it), and readily detected (most believe) by inexpensive tests (we can find it).

All newborns, incidentally, are tested for hypothyroidism by law in most places in order to prevent the condition called cretinism, which is mental retardation and short stature caused by low thyroid. Otherwise, experts disagree about who needs routine screening for hypothyroidism. The American College of Physicians recommends it for all women above fifty years of age. Men were not felt to be at enough risk to warrant routine testing, nor were younger women. The American Thyroid Association has published aggressive guidelines suggesting that men and women over thirty-five should be tested every five years. The American Academy of Family Physicians recommends screening everyone over sixty. The U.S. Department of Health and Human Services (DHHS) and the Institute of Medicine (IOM) co-funded research that concluded no screening of any kind was justified.

MY CRITERIA FOR THYROID TESTING

Do you need a thyroid check? The list below reflects my own opinion about who should be tested, but it was developed with published guidelines in mind, at least the ones formulated by those without their heads completely in the sand. This book focuses on low thyroid; therefore, I have excluded those situations in which thyroid testing should be done to rule out high levels of thyroid hormone (that is, hyperthyroidism). Among those who should be tested are:

• All women over age fifty every five years.

- Women over age thirty-five who have a family history of any thyroid disease, every three to five years.

- Men over age thirty-five who have a family history of low thyroid. A low-thyroid man often has a history of thyroid disease in female relatives. But since thyroid and autoimmune problems are rarer in men, it's not essential to screen all men in such families, provided they and their doctors remain alert for warning signs.

- All pregnant women. Maternal hypothyroidism impairs the future intellectual development of the child and must be avoided.

- Everybody with at least six of the twelve findings on the Zulewski list and perhaps everybody with at least three of them. Those with fewer than three Zulewski findings should be tested only if there are other reasons to suspect thyroid disease, such as family history or the presence of a low-thyroid feature not on the list, like chronic fatigue.

- Everybody with a major thyroid-linked disorder, such as infertility, menstrual irregularity, dyslipidemia, and psychiatric disease (especially depression).

- Everybody with a structural thyroid problem, such as a goiter or thyroid nodule(s).

- Everybody with a past thyroid problem of any kind not now being treated. Examples include persons with low (or high) levels that got better spontaneously or after past treatment, and anyone told they had a problem that was too mild to treat.

- Everybody who received destructive therapy to or near the thyroid in the past, such as thyroid surgery, radioactive iodine for high thyroid, or external-beam radiation for certain cancers, especially Hodgkin's disease.

CHAPTER 3

LOW-THYROID DIAGNOSIS

Mainstream physicians agree that the only reliable way to confirm hypothyroidism is with biochemical blood testing. The signs and symptoms of an underactive thyroid we've just discussed raise suspicion and justify further evaluation, but they do not, by themselves, nail the diagnosis.

Some reformists disagree. Don't bother with blood tests, they say. This entire book is a concession that they might be partly right, but mostly they are wrong. To completely dispense with laboratory testing would rob us of one of the four limbs of modern diagnostic evaluation: history, examination, lab tests, and imaging. Like a three-legged dog, clinical evaluation without laboratory tests gets nowhere fast (and might get hit by a car while making the effort).

Before beginning our discussion of thyroid blood testing, two categories of nonbiochemical testing deserve mention, mainly for their questionable value. The first are radiological studies—x-rays and the like —which are often ordered but have no role in the workup of pure hypothyroidism. The second is a clinical test espoused by reformists—the measurement of basal body temperature—which is either unknown to or ignored by the mainstream.

RADIOLOGY

Two imaging procedures commonly performed on the thyroid gland are ultrasound and nuclear medicine thyroid scanning. I often order both on hypothyroid patients, but never for the sole purpose of figuring out whether or why a person has low thyroid hormone levels. Ultrasound scans define anatomy (that is, size, shape, and consistency of the thyroid gland) in the evaluation of a goiter or thyroid nodule. Many hypothyroid patients have these structural abnormalities, and I often order either or both for that reason, but never specifically because of the hypothyroidism. The same is true with nuclear medicine thyroid scans—they are useful in the evaluation of nodules and *hyper*thyroidism, not hypothyroidism. Neither test is dangerous, but you owe it to your pocketbook, or your insurance company's, to ask why a thyroid ultrasound or scan is needed. If the answer involves a thyroid lump or enlargement, even if your doctor just wants to make sure you don't have one, fine. If it's just a knee-jerk reaction to a low level of thyroid hormone, it's a waste of time and money.

BASAL BODY TEMPERATURE

Basal body temperature (BBT) determination was proposed in the 1940s as a way of documenting low body temperature and hence low body metabolism. To determine BBT, a person takes his or her temperature daily, first thing in the morning, for a month, then calculates the average. It's a reasonable idea, but not something conventional doctors ever talk about or learn about. Yet some reformists swear by BBT testing, claiming that everyone with a low BBT has low thyroid, regardless of what any other finding may show.

Profoundly low thyroid levels may measurably decrease body temperature. Presumably, though, most people whose body temperatures are *that* low should be picked up with lab tests. Even if milder, less easily recognizable thyroid failure also does decrease BBT, I'm skeptical of a test that relies on home thermometers and readings taken by untrained people. Because error and uncertainty exist in all data collection, no result of any kind is worth more than the technique used to create it. The needed precision, accuracy, and quality control to make BBT a useful diagnostic tool just isn't there. Instruments purchased from a retail grocer or pharmacy will vary in quality and accuracy, and the skills with which they are employed also vary. The average mom does fine taking her child's temperature, but don't make the mistake of thinking that it's a perfect reading. It's fine for deciding if the tyke needs Tylenol or should visit the pediatrician, but it's inadequate for measuring subtle changes in cellular metabolism.

And I'll let you in on a secret—we doctors take body temperatures measured in the hospital by trained nurses with a huge grain of salt. Fevers of 102°F or 103°F catch our attention, but changes of a few tenths of a degree, even a whole degree, we don't get too excited about. Which means, rightly or wrongly, a sheet of temperature readings done at home and presented to a physician is likely to be considered just short of worthless.

My cynicism aside, even cursory research into BBT reveals problems. One reformist author says stick the thermometer in one's mouth, another in the armpit. Every first-year medical student knows that temperature readings vary widely depending on the site measured. The author who said use the mouth also said to keep the thermometer in place for two minutes. My physical exam textbook from medical school states that up to eight minutes might be required for an accurate reading. One book claimed that an average BBT of under 97.6°F (normal is 98.6°F) was evidence of hypothyroidism; some say perhaps even less than 98.0°F. My textbook, though, says that normal morning oral temperatures can fall as low as 96.4°F.

Properly done, according to a rigid protocol, there might be something to BBT testing. In its present form, though, it is not widely accepted and has not been proven valid by any scientific study I'm aware of. Even if we assume all hypothyroid patients have low BBTs—100 percent sensitivity, no false negatives (unlikely for any test)—then what about the false positives? How many reasons for a low BBT are there that have nothing to do with thyroid disease? The reformists who claim BBT testing reveals all don't talk about that.

Tribute to a Forgotten Pioneer

I recently had the pleasure of reading another description of basal temperature testing—this one authored by Broda Barnes, M.D. Like most currently practicing physicians, I was unaware of Dr. Barnes and his work prior to starting my research for *The Thyroid Paradox*. Some reformist authors hold him in godlike regard. He was the original describer, in

1942, of the BBT test, and his proclamations seem to constitute the basis for the persisting myth that thyroid blood tests are utterly worthless. With all due respect to Dr. Barnes, his work and experience date from the late 1930s and did not extend beyond the mid-1970s, when his book was published. Our major contemporary thyroid function tests hadn't been developed by then, so his comments, which may have been perfectly valid when he made them, are irrelevant today.

Nevertheless, as I read Dr. Barnes's book, *Hypothyroidism: The Unsuspected Illness* (HarperCollins, 1976), I surprised myself by agreeing with much of what it said. I came to regard my book as a much-needed update of his work. His research on basal temperature testing was published in top journals until about 1960. I suspect interest waned after that due to the rise of laboratory technology (the TSH blood test came along right about then). By the way, he recommended using a thermometer in the armpit for ten minutes to measure temperature. And he talks about sensitivity and specificity and conditions other than hypothyroidism that might cause a false-positive result. With respect to the questionable value of thyroid blood tests, I entirely agree with what he said, as far as it goes. The tests he would have dealt with—which don't include modern TSH assays—were of little value. My conclusion is that Dr. Barnes had worthy ideas that the mainstream lost track of in the past few decades. Reformists may be right in resurrecting some of them, but as they do so, I'd prefer a little more scientific circumspection.

Be warned, anybody recommending BBT testing today is coloring way outside the lines of conventional medical practice. I prefer to rely on my eyes, ears, brain, and a healthy skepticism of nonetheless well-validated blood tests. If you're determined to do a BBT test, there's no harm in it. But before you spend a month gathering data, make sure your doctor is willing to look at it and has some idea of what to do with it. Most won't and you'll be disappointed.

THYROID BLOOD TESTS

Diagnosis and treatment of low thyroid are irrevocably linked. What we are trying to diagnose is thyroid disease needing treatment. The question, then, is less "How do we diagnose low thyroid?" and more "How do we decide whom to treat?" That distinction might not be crystal clear, so let's expand upon it. If thyroid tests are abnormal, we make a diagnosis, right? And if we make a diagnosis, we treat it, right? Not necessarily on either count. Later, we'll have a discussion about what "normal" means. For now, normal is normal. And I'll stipulate that if a test result is abnormal, we have a diagnosis. But diagnosis does not equal initiating treatment. Whether or not treatment should be started depends on the severity of the problem versus how cheap, easy, and painless the cure is. For any test, the level of abnormality that must be reached before a physician actually does anything about it is called its "treatment threshold."

Thyrotropin or Thyroid-Stimulating Hormone (TSH) Test

The most frequently ordered thyroid-function test is measurement of the serum level of thyrotropin or thyroid-stimulating hormone (TSH), which costs about fifty dollars. If you only get one thyroid test, this is usually the one you want. Remember, TSH is the pituitary secretion that regulates the thyroid gland. As thyroid hormone levels rise in the blood, TSH levels fall, and vice versa. Assays to measure this hormone have existed since 1964, and by the 1980s had improved to the point of becoming the single best indicator of thyroid status, high or low, according to most experts.

Rightly or wrongly, TSH is *the* test upon which most thyroid treatment decisions are made today, decisions about starting therapy as well as about adjusting it. If you and your doctor are serious about getting to the bottom of what's going on with your thyroid, and you haven't had your TSH checked, demand it—after you consider finding a more up-to-date doctor. Overall, I agree that the TSH test is the single best thyroid function test. The operative word is *single*. By itself, it's the best of the lot. No expert, however, believes TSH alone can diagnose all thyroid abnormalities. Most, perhaps, but not all.

What makes the TSH test superior to other thyroid tests? First, production of TSH by the pituitary responds briskly to small changes in thyroid hormone levels in the blood. A minuscule decrease in thyroxine

(T_4) exponentially elevates TSH. That means TSH sets off alarms about a low-thyroid situation early, often while thyroxine and triiodothyronine (T_3) levels still appear normal. Statistically speaking, TSH is more sensitive for thyroid failure than other blood chemistries. TSH is a fishing net rather than a pole.

Assays of TSH also indicate tissue thyroid levels more accurately than alternative tests. Effectively, they mine below the surface of thyroid system physiology. When tests measure T_4 or T_3 levels in the blood, that's all we get—levels in the blood. What we really want to know is if enough thyroid hormone is getting deep into the brain, heart, skeletal muscles, and so forth. TSH also gives us a peek inside that black box, described in Chapter 1, where deiodinases convert inactive T_4 to active T_3. That's because TSH release is governed by T_3 in the brain and pituitary, much of which comes from deiodinase-driven peripheral conversion.

So, TSH is more sensitive and comprehensive than other tests. It evaluates all levels of thyroid regulation, from the brain and the pituitary gland, to the thyroid gland, and to tissues throughout the body. Within limits, it measures global thyroid system function. What are those limits? The way most doctors use TSH testing, it's clear they assume the link between pituitary TSH secretion and thyroid T_4 secretion to be forged in iron. For them, for every x elevation of TSH, T_4 always goes up y. For every y decrease in T_4, TSH always goes up x. They also assume that the tissue effects of thyroid hormone are equally intense inside and outside the central nervous system.

There are times when one or both of those assumptions don't hold. The linkage between TSH and thyroid hormone can be broken or damaged so that TSH does not go up as it should when thyroid levels drop. The brain sometimes gets more or less thyroid effect than the rest of the body, meaning it might inaccurately interpret the body's needs. Either scenario can screw up the thyroid system in a way that TSH testing alone might give no clue about. With one exception—central hypothyroidism—this chapter will not cover those oddball situations. For now, we continue to view the world through rose-colored glasses, a world in which lab tests tell all and, like George Washington, cannot tell a lie.

Normal and Abnormal TSH Levels

As with all blood tests, the range of TSH values considered normal varies with the individual laboratory, but it's generally in the neighborhood of 0.3–5.0 milliunits per liter (mU/L). Remember, though, we care less about whether TSH is normal than we do about whether it is above or below treatment threshold—that point above which TSH indicates hypothyroidism serious enough to do something about.

Guidelines endorsed by two organizations—the American College of Physicians and the American Association of Clinical Endocrinologists—support offering therapy if TSH climbs above 10.0 mU/L. What about a TSH less strikingly abnormal, for instance, between 5.0 and 10.0 mU/L? This is a muddled gray zone. Everybody agrees that it's not normal, but does it need fixing? The American College of Physicians leans toward no treatment, with repeat testing in a few years. An article in *Thyroid*, the American Thyroid Association's journal, essentially echoed this recommendation. The American Association of Clinical Endocrinologists takes a more aggressive approach: they support treatment for a TSH of 5.0–10.0 mU/L in patients if they have a goiter or positive thyroid antibody tests.

In the 2003 film *Pirates of the Caribbean: The Curse of the Black Pearl*, a running joke was that the Pirates' Code was really "more of a guideline." The same is true of recommendations from organizations like the American College of Physicians and American Association of Clinical Endocrinologists. They're guidelines, not hard-and-fast laws. They tend to be conservative, avoiding treatment where possible. That's the safe approach under a "first, do no harm" paradigm. Plus, guidelines have to be broad enough to cover many situations. They are like the average of a set of numbers. Similarly, some perfectly reputable doctors will be more aggressive than the guidelines suggest, others will be more cautious.

I am a mainstream endocrinologist whose management of hypothyroidism falls on the aggressive side. I definitely agree with giving thyroid pills to almost all people with a TSH exceeding 10.0 mU/L. As for the mildly abnormal group—TSH between 5.0 and 10.0—I usually treat, provided the patient agrees after I explain the controversies. My rationale is that thyroid replacement is relatively cheap and safe. With little cost or risk, I can prevent worsening hypothyroidism in the future. Not everyone gets worse if not treated, though; some people improve on their own. Naysayers cite this as justification for doing nothing. It is possible, to some extent, to predict the future. People with certain positive antibody tests, for example, progress to full-blown hypothyroidism about twice as often as those without.

Two reasons for treating mild (so-called subclinical) hypothyroidism are to prevent future problems and to help existing ones. And while I'm all for the first reason, I treat most people with a TSH above 5.0 mU/L for the second, to help them now. My patient's risk of getting worse is secondary, if she needs relief from something already bothering her. So, the $64,000 question is: Is mild hypothyroidism a bad thing? Bad enough to treat?

Uncertainty exists, but research suggests that correction of mild thyroid deficiency may lower the risk of heart attack and stroke, improve dyslipidemia, and prevent or improve depression. Many people also simply feel better on thyroid hormone. One paper, whose authors reviewed many

---

Key Points about TSH Testing for Low Thyroid

- TSH is the most sensitive single test.

- TSH rises greatly with slight drops in T_4 or T_3.

- *High* TSH indicates *low* thyroid (this confuses many people).

- TSH estimates both tissue and blood thyroid hormone levels.

- The normal range for TSH, in most labs, is up to about 5.0 mU/L.

- Most doctors treat people with a TSH greater than 10.0 mU/L.

- Some doctors treat people with a TSH greater than 5.0 mU/L.

- Sometimes TSH fails to rise despite hypothyroidism.

studies on the subject, concluded that patients with a TSH in the 5.0–10.0 mU/L range were more likely to show poor heart function than those with a normal TSH. That paper recommended a treatment threshold of 4.0 mU/L or greater. My own TSH, by the way, was 7.5 mU/L before I started on thyroid hormone pills. So, for what it's worth, I'm not recommending anything I don't do myself.

The Problem of Central Hypothyroidism

Many conscientious doctors assess thyroid status with TSH tests alone. After all, they've been taught that it's the single best test. There are circumstances, though, where true low-thyroid patients do not have high TSH levels. This occurs when there is damage to the pituitary gland or parts of the brain that regulate it. If the hypothalamus can't make enough thyrotropin-releasing hormone (TRH) and/or the pituitary can't make enough TSH, then the thyroid won't make enough thyroid hormone. This is called central hypothyroidism. (Regular hypothyroidism, in which the problem is theoretically limited to the thyroid gland itself, is called *primary* hypothyroidism.) Patients with central hypothyroidism have the same clinical findings as those with primary hypothyroidism, but TSH will be low or normal. It could be slightly high, but lower than it should be, considering the severity of thyroid hormone deficiency. Often the only clues to central hypothyroidism are found in the patient's history, examination, or actual T_4 or T_3 levels. If a TSH test alone is ordered and the clinical evaluation is inadequate or ignored, central hypothyroidism can easily be missed.

To avoid this, I usually get at least one other thyroid blood test along with the TSH test. Sometimes, by the way, a high TSH level is seen in a hyperthyroid (high-thyroid) patient. This is very rare, but I mention it for completeness and to further illustrate the pitfalls of a TSH-only approach to thyroid evaluation.

The foregoing discussion shows that rules are made to be broken, even in the well-ordered world of mainstream endocrinology. That will be our battle cry moving forward. First, though, we have more tests to explore.

Free Thyroxine/Free T$_4$ Test

After the TSH level, the next best blood test for hypothyroidism is generally considered to be the free thyroxine (FT$_4$) test. This assay is one way of measuring how much T$_4$ (the most abundant product of the thyroid gland) is in the blood. In relatively severe hypothyroidism, FT$_4$ is low and TSH is high. That's the classic pattern of primary hypothyroidism. In milder cases, though, FT$_4$ is often normal despite a high TSH. In other words, as the thyroid gland fails, TSH rises before FT$_4$ falls. Compared to TSH, FT$_4$ is less sensitive but more specific. A fishing pole, not a net.

"Free" refers to that portion of T$_4$ swimming loose in the blood. Only this so-called free fraction can enter target cells and be turned into T$_3$ or otherwise trigger some thyroid hormone effect. At least, that's what most of us assume based on the "free hormone hypothesis." Something like 99.98 percent of all blood T$_4$ is bound, not free. By bound, I mean T$_4$ molecules that are chained to serum transport proteins like galley slaves as they circulate through the body. Bound T$_4$ can't do anything; therefore, free T$_4$ measures only that small percentage of thyroid hormone that is ready and able to work, which, in theory, is all we care about.

It is difficult and expensive for laboratories to physically separate free T$_4$ from bound T$_4$, so only a few actually do that. Most T$_4$ tests are estimates of the free fraction, rather than direct measures of it. Sometimes these estimates come from two separate tests: one to measure T$_4$ and one to measure transport proteins. The results are factored together using simple arithmetic. The two-step test is called a free thyroxine index (see below).

The FT$_4$ test discussed here refers to any single-test method of estimating the free fraction of thyroxine in the blood. In practice, we consider these superior to two-step methods, but the FT$_4$ is still just an estimate. And "estimate" should translate in your mind to "inaccurate." Perhaps not dismally so, but in some common situations, like pregnancy, the FT$_4$ can be downright wrong. And in the best of situations, FT$_4$ is still less sensitive for detecting low thyroid than TSH.

For these reasons, the National Academy of Clinical Biochemistry advises not to use the free T_4 test alone to assess thyroid function. They recommend either a TSH alone, or a free T_4 estimate plus a TSH test. Being a pole not a net, FT_4 alone misses too many low-thyroid cases. That said, if your FT_4 *is* low—below the laboratory's published normal range— you probably need treatment. Free T_4 is great for ruling *in* disease, just not so good at ruling it *out*.

Some labs do what they call a reflex FT_4. They automatically measure FT_4 if the TSH is abnormal. That gets the benefits of two tests—a net and a pole—and avoids the cost of running both on everybody. However, the reflex method might still miss central hypothyroidism. For that reason, the FT_4 test must be run regardless of TSH when there are reasons to suspect pituitary or hypothalamus problems (a history of tumor or surgery in those areas, for instance, or any head trauma). This is an example of why laboratory tests should never be interpreted without clinical information.

Total Thyroxine/Total T_4 Test

The free T_4 test measures the approximately 0.02 percent of T_4 not clinging to serum transport proteins. The total thyroxine (TT_4) test measures, unsurprisingly, everything. It measures T_4 that is both bound to protein and free in the blood. The TT_4 is cheaper than FT_4 and more laboratories can run a TT_4 on site, meaning doctors get results faster. But perhaps the biggest reason that the TT_4 is still used is habit. It's an older test—in my opinion, obsolete—but more doctors are accustomed to it and we're a pretty stubborn bunch.

What's the problem? TT_4 is cheaper, faster, and more familiar—all good things. Unfortunately, it doesn't measure what we want to know. We want to know how much thyroid hormone is getting to where the action is. If some test reads abnormal, but the thyroid still gets the job done— that is, the patient doesn't have tissue hypothyroidism—then what difference does it make? FT_4 is bad enough. It purports to show what's available to tissues, instead of what's accomplished within them. TT_4 is another step backward, because more than 99 percent of what it measures is sequestered by transport proteins. It represents the stockpile available to replenish the "worker bee" hormones, but says nothing about the worker bee faction itself.

To manage thyroid disease with TT_4 alone is like a general leading a battle knowing how many troops he has in reserve, but not how many are on the front lines. At best, TT_4 is a crude estimate of FT_4—which itself is only an estimate. Are you getting the picture that thyroid function testing isn't an exact science? This is something doctors should also keep in mind when deciding whether to treat patients or numbers.

Total T_4 would work as a fast, cheap estimate of FT_4 if the ratio between the total and free fractions was equal in everybody, but it isn't. It doesn't even stay the same in a single person over time. When the level of thyroxine-binding globulin (TBG), the main transport protein, increases, so does TT_4. More boats, more galley slaves. But the amount of free hormone doesn't change. So, depending on how much TBG there is, the ratio of total hormone to free hormone varies. And all sorts of things affect TBG levels, including pregnancy, liver disease, and a number of drugs. Estrogen is a common culprit: women on birth control pills or taking postmenopausal hormone replacement may have a high TT_4 solely due to estrogen. TBG drops with malnutrition and kidney failure and in those taking steroids, testosterone, and certain epilepsy drugs.

Here's one of the few times you'll catch me saying "always" or "never" about a medical topic. I *never* willingly order only a TT_4 when trying to make a new diagnosis of hypothyroidism. Statistically, TT_4 is at least as insensitive as FT_4 and it is less specific. Its rates of false positives and false negatives are high. I doubt there is any place in the United States where you can't get a TSH in short order, and all insurance plans should cover it. Nevertheless, some doctors still order the TT_4 alone to screen for thyroid disease, a diagnostic strategy I consider next to worthless. If you've been told "It's not your thyroid" and the only thyroid test done was a TT_4, get further testing.

Out of respect for the open-minded questioning of scientific dogma, I feel compelled to add something before continuing. All the positive things I've said about free T_4 tests and the negative things about total T_4 tests assume the correctness of the free hormone hypothesis—that it is the free fraction and not the bound fraction of thyroid hormone that does most of the work in the body. Later, though, I'll mention research suggesting that transport proteins might have a key role in delivering thyroid hormone to individual cells. If so, total T_4 tests may actually be a better reflection of what's available to tissues than free T_4 tests. (There are different and firmly valid reasons to prefer TSH over TT_4 testing in most situations. It's the supposed superiority of FT_4 over TT_4 at issue here.) I don't know the answer, but I hope it will eventually be proven that we (the mainstream) have been more right than wrong all this time. Meanwhile, we definitely need to be more humble in the face of all we don't know.

T_3-Resin Uptake

If the total T_4 test is so inept, how did we muddle through before free T_4 tests became affordable and readily available, which was only in the mid-1990s or so? The previous discussion was about TT_4 flying solo. There is a difficult-to-comprehend test, the bane of medical students, called the T_3-resin uptake (T_3RU)—also known as the T_3 uptake or thyroid hormone–binding ratio (THBR)—which is designed to help the TT_4. The T_3RU test has caused more confusion than any test I know of. First, it is *not* a measure of serum triiodothyronine (T_3); even doctors routinely make that mistake. Suffice it to say, T_3RU is a fudge factor: it measures the impact of changes in transport protein (TBG) levels on TT_4 and corrects for them.

Most of the time, the T_3RU test actually works. A common circumstance where it doesn't is during a severe illness or trauma, in response to which the body produces chemicals that interfere with binding to TBG. This may be more than coincidence. Perhaps it is advantageous to reduce the pool of T_4 available to sick cells struggling on meager resources. Maybe reduced thyroid hormone, resulting in reduced metabolism, is the body putting itself to bed and slurping chicken soup for a while.

The point is, in severe illness, the T_3RU test isn't smart enough to tell low TBG binding from low TBG levels. Both TT_4 and T_3RU plunge as a result, producing a pattern of numbers the unwary doctor might mistake for hypothyroidism. However, in this case, the person's thyroid system is normal and the changes are solely a consequence of severe nonthyroid illness. We call this situation euthyroid sick syndrome. If the doctor then treats the nonexistent low-thyroid condition, the already overtaxed body might become further stressed, resulting in harm.

Free Thyroxine Index

The free thyroxine index (FTI) is an estimate of the free fraction of thyroxine calculated using a mathematical formula into which values for TT_4 and T_3RU are plugged. This is the two-step estimate of free T_4 mentioned above. Most laboratories offer a set of studies called a thyroid panel, consisting of a TT_4 test, a T_3RU test, and a calculated FTI. If the FTI is normal, it's usually okay to ignore the other two tests, normal or otherwise.

Here's a pearl of wisdom: if TT_4 and T_3RU are abnormal in the same direction, it probably indicates a real problem; if they're abnormal in opposite directions—one high, one low—it probably indicates a transport protein problem that doesn't require treatment.

The FTI is often an adequate substitute for a FT_4. They are both, however, only estimates of what we want to know and both are susceptible to protein-binding confusion. Frankly, their performance is probably not as different as is often thought. Nevertheless, I consider the TT_4 and T_3RU, and anything convolutedly derived from them, to be obsolete. Under the best of conditions, any blood test is going to be wrong some percentage of the time. Since the FTI depends on two separate tests, the risk of it being wrong is the sum of the error rates of both tests—this is certainly a case where two wrongs don't make a right.

Many doctors still use the thyroid panel and calculated FTI, but I don't recommend accepting a diagnosis of "Your thyroid's normal" until at least a TSH and a one-step FT_4 have been done. For most patients—pregnant women being a prominent exception—I simply don't have sufficient faith in the FTI.

Total and Free Triiodothyronine (T₃)

Much of what has already been said about T_4 tests also applies to serum triiodothyronine (T_3) measurement tests. The only real difference is that the free fraction of T_3 is about 0.2 percent of the total, tenfold greater than the free fraction of T_4. Tests of T_3, therefore, are less affected by TBG changes, but they are still affected. That is, a total T_3 (TT_3) test by itself is not as worthless as a TT_4. Nevertheless, many lean toward using free T_3 (FT_3) levels for the same reasons we prefer the FT_4 test. Some experts, though, advise against trusting the accuracy of FT_3 measurements. Bottom line: either a free or total T_3 is fine, provided it is recognized that both are mere estimates, subject to errors and interference. They need to be interpreted thoughtfully in view of other lab tests and the clinical status of the individual.

A greater question looms about serum T_3 testing: Should we do it at all? For mainstream doctors—despite its unquestioned vital role in the thyroid system—T_3 is the poor hormonal stepsister of T_4. T_4 is the star of thyroid evaluation because it is abundant and levels remain fairly stable hour to hour and day to day. Normal blood levels of T_3 are about fifty times lower than T_4, making it harder to measure, and it has a shorter life span in the blood, making it less stable. Levels may change from, say, morning to afternoon, so the tests are harder to interpret. If a woman's FT_3 is lower today than three months ago, the question is: Is she more hypothyroid or was the blood drawn at a different time of day? Also, T_3 testing (compared to T_4) is done by far fewer laboratories.

Now, just because the current state of the art adores T_4 and shuns T_3 doesn't mean we have to. Reformists tend to champion T_3 as the holy grail of thyroid testing and that point of view is easy to justify. If T_3 is the more potent hormone, and the actual molecule infiltrating the target cell's nucleus and mating with its chromosome-bound receptor, then shouldn't we be measuring it instead of T_4? Yes, but we're back to that black box problem. If we had a practical test for T_3 inside the nuclei of cells, I'd be on board—but we don't. All we can measure is blood T_3, which may bear little, if any, resemblance to what's happening behind closed doors, a few microns over, in the cell. Worse, in all but the most severe cases of hypothyroidism, T_3 production actually increases! Deiodinase converts more of what T_4 there is into T_3. As a result, conventional thyroidological wisdom is that T_3 not only is *not* the best indicator of a low-thyroid state, it may have no meaning at all.

Thyroid Antibody Testing

Thyroid antibody testing is done relatively infrequently compared to the other thyroid blood tests. When it is done, it usually doesn't add much. Antibodies are composed of complex proteins called immunoglobulins. With few exceptions, normal antibodies are produced as a reaction to the body's exposure to a foreign particle, such as an influenza bug. The attached antibody acts like a tag, flagging the invading object for demolition by the immune system. An autoantibody, however, is any immunoglobulin that binds inappropriately to a target belonging to one's own body. Finding autoantibodies in the blood may indicate the presence of an autoimmune disease.

Most thyroid disorders are autoimmune in origin. Thus, tests for thyroid autoantibodies are done as a screen for the presence of autoimmune thyroid disease. There are three main thyroid antibody tests: antithyroid peroxidase antibodies, anti-thyroglobulin antibodies, and TSH-receptor antibodies. To elaborate:

• Antithyroid peroxidase antibodies (TPOAbs) attack specific structures inside the thyroid follicular cell. TPOAb tests are positive in many thyroid disorders and can be thought of as a general flag for thyroid disease. If present at very high levels, TPOAbs are diagnostic for Hashimoto's thyroiditis, the autoimmune disease considered to be the most common spontaneous cause of hypothyroidism.

• Anti-thyroglobulin antibodies attack the protein thyroglobulin. Testing for them reveals nothing the TPOAb test doesn't cover, so I don't order this test by itself. Its only real use is to confirm the validity of a serum thyroglobulin level, which is used mostly to monitor thyroid cancer. This antibody test has no role in the workup of someone who may be hypothyroid.

• TSH-receptor antibodies (thyroid-stimulating immunoglobulins or TSIs) are the root cause of Graves' disease, the most common cause of hyperthyroidism. They are of no significance in the diagnosis of low thyroid. They will crop up later, though, as a confounder in the treatment of the hypothyroidism that often follows Graves' disease.

With respect to initially evaluating a low-thyroid state, TPOAb is the only antibody test that is conceivably useful. A hypothyroid patient with high TPOAb levels probably has Hashimoto's thyroiditis. It is rarely important, however, to know what caused a person's hypothyroidism, because the treatment is the same regardless—thyroid hormone pills. (Hardcore reformists will have a problem with that statement. Often they insist on fixing the underlying problem with, for example, nutritional therapy. That's a nice idea, but in the mainstream world there is currently no proven way to do that.) If you really must know, the cause of a particular case of low thyroid will either be obvious—surgery or radioactive iodine treatment—or it's probably Hashimoto's thyroiditis. There really is no need to bother with antibody testing in the diagnosis of hypothyroidism.

A common reason endocrinologists do order TPOAb tests is to decide about, not diagnosis, but treatment. Specifically, what to do about a TSH in the 5.0–10.0 mU/L range. Remember, such results indicate mild hypothyroidism for which there is controversy over the need for treatment. A mildly high TSH that is accompanied by an elevated TPOAb is more likely to worsen than is one that is not accompanied by elevated antibodies. If your doctor is a cautious type who doesn't believe in treating all mild hypothyroidism, then a positive TPOAb may tip the scale toward treatment. At the very least, anybody with a high TPOAb needs frequent testing and examination. I treat virtually everybody with a high TSH, regardless of how high, so I don't often feel the need to order a TPOAb. If I have a reluctant patient, however, a positive TPOAb might help me convince her to proceed with treatment.

Antibody testing is a minor point of disagreement between mainstreamists and reformists. Certain reformists believe antibody testing to be *the* way of identifying folks with normal thyroid levels who might be truly hypothyroid. I don't wholeheartedly disagree, but I differ in how I think the information should be used. If a TPOAb test is positive in a patient whose thyroid tests and clinical evaluation are otherwise normal, I would say she is at risk of low thyroid and needs to be watched. A reformist might say she has low thyroid and proceed with treatment.

TRH Stimulation Test

The last test we'll discuss is not one you can walk into a lab and have accomplished with a simple blood draw. It is a procedure performed in the office of an experienced physician, usually an endocrinologist. The hypothalamus, located at the center of the brain, produces thyrotropin-releasing hormone (TRH). TRH stimulates the pituitary to make TSH, which stimulates the thyroid to make T_4 and T_3. The whole system, the hypothalamic-pituitary-thyroid (HPT) axis, is under negative-feedback control. Increasing T_4 and T_3 levels lower TRH and TSH, which leads to decreased T_4 and T_3; this then stimulates TSH and TRH to again increase T_4 and T_3, starting the cycle over again.

Testing blood levels of T_4 directly evaluates the thyroid, and TSH levels directly test pituitary function. The TRH stimulation test (TRH test or TRH-stim test) evaluates the entire HPT axis. Some reformists—those who haven't completely rejected blood testing—are fans of TRH testing as a means of finding hidden thyroid abnormalities. Some mainstreamists believe the procedure to be obsolete. I and most endocrinologists fall somewhere in the middle.

TRH stimulation is an example of dynamic endocrine testing. When endocrinologists think a hormone is low, they try to stimulate its production. If they can't, they conclude the gland in question is failing. If a hormone is thought to be high, on the other hand, they try to suppress it. If they can't, overproduction is diagnosed. Stimulation and suppression tests are the endocrinologist's expertise, and bread and butter.

The TRH test evaluates pituitary obedience to commands from the brain. A specially trained nurse starts an intravenous line and injects the drug Thyrel (generic name, protirelin), which is identical to human TRH.

It is safe, though a moment of nausea, urge to urinate, flushing, anxiety, or other symptoms may occur. At specific times—usually just before the injection and thirty and sixty minutes after the shot—the nurse will draw blood to measure TSH levels. Since TRH sparks the release of TSH, the normal result of a TRH injection is a doubling to quadrupling of the TSH level. If the stimulated TSH level exceeds four times the baseline level, the patient has primary hypothyroidism. A failing thyroid doesn't provide enough negative feedback, thus revving up pituitary TSH production.

If the TSH response to the injection is flat—no increase—hyperthyroidism is generally diagnosed, because excess thyroid hormone inhibits pituitary TSH production. If the response is not flat, but the peak TSH is less than twice the pre-injection level, we call this a blunted TRH response. The pituitary reacts weakly to orders from the brain, indicating a sick pituitary gland—that is, central hypothyroidism. Another possibility is brain damage in the hypothalamus. Like a fire dying from lack of being stoked, the sluggish but otherwise undamaged pituitary may still respond to TRH, but that response may be delayed, with a peak at sixty instead of thirty minutes. This finding, too, is lumped under the term *central hypothyroidism*.

So, depending on whether the TSH response to the TRH shot is high, normal, low, late, or nonexistent, we draw different conclusions about the health of the HPT axis. This is complicated, so let's recap:

• TSH increases two- to fourfold, with peak at thirty minutes after shot = Normal HPT axis

• TSH increases greater than fourfold = Sick thyroid/primary hypothyroidism

• TSH increases less than twofold = Sick pituitary or hypothalamus/central hypothyroidism

• TSH doesn't change = Overactive thyroid or severe central hypothyroidism

• TSH increases two- to fourfold with peak delayed to sixty minutes = Sick hypothalamus/central hypothyroidism

Those who declare TRH testing obsolete are saying they believe all thyroid disease can be diagnosed with serum TSH, T_4, and possibly, T_3 levels. As discussed, this is not always true. TRH testing is helpful when laboratory abnormalities are subtle or when the usual link between TSH and thyroid hormone production is broken. The latter certainly occurs in central hypothyroidism. Later, we'll look at other situations where TSH levels may not reflect true thyroid status.

Before leaving TRH testing, I should mention one huge problem with it. In July 2002, the domestic United States' production of Thyrel was halted by the manufacturer, under a mandate from, I presume, the U.S Food and Drug Administration. Therefore, as of this writing, TRH testing is not routinely available in the United States. A speaker mentioned this at a meeting I attended and an audience member, an endocrinologist from Europe, expressed shock: "What do you mean TRH isn't available?" We can put a man on the moon, but I can't do a TRH test in my office. I asked a pharmacist friend to look into this and he couldn't find anybody who knew anything and somebody in Canada hung up on him. I find it doubly odd that nobody in my field is making any noise, in speech or in print. Several Internet searches I've done fail to explain what the problem with Thyrel was. TRH testing, it seems, has vanished off the face of modern thyroidology.

Were I prone to conspiracy theories, I'd be working overtime on this one, because the TRH test was a way out of the quagmire. Until it returns—if it returns—a valuable tool is lost to thyroidologists and thyroid patients. I have significantly modified my practice as a result. Since I can't clarify borderline situations with TRH testing anymore, I'm prescribing more trials of thyroid hormone pills. In other words, testing for low thyroid by seeing if therapy helps. A technique I would have scoffed at before, and something the hardcore mainstreamist would condemn and no doubt the reformist would cheer.

CURRENT MAINSTREAM STANDARDS

We have now covered the usual methods for finding hypothyroidism needing treatment. Next, we'll discuss how conventional thyroidology can miss true hypothyroidism and how those leaks can be plugged. Before moving on, though, let's summarize the current standards of care for the diagnosis and treatment of low thyroid. I am presenting here my understanding of mainstream opinion, not necessarily my personal one. That comes later.

- History and examination are crucial to diagnosis, but no one should be treated for low thyroid without blood test confirmation of disease.

- The best single hypothyroidism test is a serum thyrotropin or thyroid-stimulating hormone (TSH) level. Any patient of any age with symptoms or signs of hypothyroidism should be evaluated with at least a TSH test.

- A screening TSH test may be reasonable even without suspicion in some people. Women older than fifty and pregnant women are at highest risk for hypothyroidism and should be tested. Some feel all men and women older than thirty-five should be screened.

- An FT_4 (free thyroxine) test or thyroid panel—total T_4 (TT_4) test, T_3-resin uptake (T_3RU), and free thyroxine index (FTI)—should be run along with the initial TSH test or used as a follow-up test if the TSH is abnormal. In general, therapy for a high TSH (indicating hypothyroidism) should be delayed until the T_4 level is confirmed to be normal or low, but not high.

- Serum T_3 tests have little, if any, place in low-thyroid evaluation.

- Most patients with a TSH greater than 10.0 mU/L should be treated. Most patients with a TSH less than 5.0 mU/L should not be treated. Patients with a TSH of 5.0–10.0 mU/L may or may not need treatment. (Endocrinologists generally treat, nonspecialists often will not.)

- Patients with goiters, thyroid nodule(s), or TPOAbs (antithyroid peroxidase antibodies) probably should be treated.

- If FT_4 or FTI test results are low, or low thyroid is otherwise strongly suspected, and the TSH is *not* greater than 5.0 mU/L, a TRH stimulation test should be done to rule out central hypothyroidism (not available in the United States as of this writing).

CHAPTER 4

HUMAN ERROR
IN THYROID TESTING

You've got a number of symptoms that could suggest hypothyroidism and decide to visit Dr. Whitecoat, bringing along a meticulously prepared list of complaints, perhaps bolstered by a book like this one, and plead for a thyroid check. He kindly complies and a few days later you get a call from the nurse: "Your thyroid levels are fine. The doctor will see you again next year."

"But, but . . ."

What is the multi-symptomatic patient to do? First, you should consider the possibility that Dr. Whitecoat is correct. Your thyroid system might be normal. In that case, your doctor should explore other explanations for your symptoms. For every medical complaint, there is a list of possible causes called its differential diagnosis. Hypothyroidism is in the differential diagnosis of fatigue, as are many other things, which may or may not be medical in nature. I see patients—often women—whose lives are quite obviously exhausting: kids, their activities, job, housework, and invalid elderly relatives all vying for their time and energy. And some people I see are saddled with still more stressful ordeals on top of the routine ones: divorce, domestic abuse, death, suicide, layoffs, even livestock plagues. Yet it seems a shock to them—absurd, even—that "life" might cause their fatigue. My point is, be frank with yourself. There is not always a disease to explain physical symptoms or always a pill to fix them.

Later, I'll give my view on the unhealthiness of stress, and specifically, its detrimental effects on the brain and endocrine system. Here's a sneak peek: if you're insisting it's your thyroid and your doctor says, "No, it's stress," you both might be right. Stress may be killing your thyroid.

Back to Dr. Whitecoat. Maybe he was right and maybe he wasn't. Perhaps it *is* your thyroid and the blip just didn't show up on his radar screen. The three ways a doctor can miss true hypothyroidism are (1) standards of care for thyroid evaluation aren't followed, (2) standards of care that underdiagnose hypothyroidism are followed, and (3) available technology misses subtle and unusual forms of hypothyroidism. In other words:

- Faulty doctor

- Faulty standards

- Faulty tests

At this point, we will address the faulty doctor factor.

SIX COMMON BLUNDERS

If Dr. Whitecoat's workup of your possible thyroid problem did not live up to the expectations outlined in the last chapter—expectations deliberately set at noncontroversial levels—you should bring your concerns to his or her attention and request more testing. Keep in mind that standards of care represent a middle ground agreed upon by most physicians. The devil is in the details. A good doctor doesn't necessarily have to follow my opinions (or those of any other physician) precisely, but a good doctor should be willing to discuss alternative approaches and/or acknowledge any weaknesses in his or her knowledge of and experience with thyroid disease. You might at this point consider seeking a second opinion, perhaps from an endocrinologist if you're not already seeing one. Don't worry—a conscientious physician should welcome the additional input. Second opinions are an integral part of the business.

The following are six common mistakes I see leading to missed diagnoses of hypothyroidism. The same list could be applied to patients on thyroid pills whose doses are left at too low a level.

History or Exam Ignored in Favor of Test Results

Biochemical testing is usually a better indicator of thyroid status than clinical evaluation, but if someone looks and sounds hypothyroid, normal test results should be eyed with suspicion. If it looks like a duck and quacks like a duck, it might *be* a duck, even if some piece of paper says it's a guinea hen. In other words, a good doctor should always entertain the possible significance of clinical signs and symptoms, regardless of what conclusion is supported by laboratory test results.

TSH Test Is Not Done

Fortunately, this problem occurs less and less often, but any initial thyroid workup that consists of only a T_4 or T_3 test doesn't hold water. There are situations where TSH is inaccurate or where it's okay to skip TSH testing, but almost never in a patient being newly evaluated. Most of the time, a TSH level is an essential component of low thyroid testing.

Failure to Treat a High TSH Simply Because T_4 or T_3 Tests Are Normal

Whether or not to treat subclinical hypothyroidism—defined as a high TSH with normal T_4 and T_3 levels—is a legitimate controversy in thyroidology today. The mistake is in not even considering therapy or recognizing the controversy. Too often, primary-care providers let other normal tests completely obviate the finding of a high TSH. That is not reasonable if we acknowledge the superior sensitivity (positivity in disease) of TSH over other thyroid function tests, which have much higher false-negative rates (that is, low sensitivity). In hypothyroidism, when tests disagree, TSH is usually the one that's right. This is especially true for high TSH levels, which are rarely wrong.

Blowing Off a TSH of 5.0–10.0 mU/L as Insignificant or Not Warranting Therapy

This sounds the same as the last "mistake" on our list, but there is a subtle distinction. In the last instance, I had in mind a doctor failing to see any pathology in a set of thyroid tests with only one abnormality showing up. Here, I'm picturing a doctor who is fully aware that a mildly high TSH (regardless of T_4 or T_3 levels) indicates mild thyroid deficiency, and yet he or she blindly adheres to recommendations saying that this degree of hypothyroidism should not be treated. Granted, there is no universal agreement about treating mild TSH elevation (subclinical hypothyroidism), but if a patient's TSH is even a little high and she has complaints that could be related to low thyroid, I think it's wrong not to offer a trial of thyroid hormone pills. At the very least, the patient with this problem should be referred to a specialist for further consideration. What are doctors trying to prove when they deny treatment to a patient who has persistent symptoms suggestive of a disease and whose test data is at least mildly consistent with the same disease?

Failure to Retest Borderline Results

Not everybody with slightly abnormal thyroid function tests needs therapy, but those who aren't treated should at least be monitored periodically to make sure the problem doesn't persist or worsen. Even if the numbers don't change, the development of a new goiter (enlarged thyroid gland) or the appearance of thyroid nodules might justify giving thyroid pills.

Failure to Consider Central Hypothyroidism

It is wrong not to consider a brain or pituitary gland problem when the TSH is normal or low, and the patient has other evidence of thyroid lack, either clinical or biochemical. In my experience, this possibility is in few doctors' differential diagnosis of thyroid-like complaints. Central hypothyroidism is said to be rare compared to primary hypothyroidism. Rare, however, doesn't mean nonexistent and it might be more common than most believe. Central hypothyroidism especially must be entertained when there is any history of trauma, surgery, or disease involving the head. And under the trauma category, something as seemingly insignificant as a mild concussion from a fall, assault, or traffic accident might qualify.

FAILURE OF INTERPRETATION

This is the "faulty standards" factor listed above. That is, a doctor can conscientiously follow the protocol outlined at the end of the last chapter and still miss hypothyroidism. Not because the tests are technically flawed (we'll deal with that issue later), but because the way we have chosen to decipher them is. It's hard to fault doctors on this one. They're following the rules, and doing what they were taught by respected mentors. Rules, however, with respect to thyroid disease, were made to be broken. More reading between the lines of blood test reports is needed. The answers may not always appear in black and white.

I have the utmost respect for the generalist's breadth of knowledge and experience. But perhaps it's unfair to expect the average primary-care provider to read between these lines. It's a little like asking the corner filling station mechanic to work on a Ferrari. He might be able to pull it off with a good enough manual, but you wouldn't want him experimenting. You'd want him to do just what the book says—no less, and certainly no more.

Like the specialty mechanic, an endocrinologist may feel more comfortable coloring outside the lines with a hormone problem than a primary-care doctor would. One of the biggest differences between specialists and generalists is their interpretation of test data. Primary-care providers are more likely to accept the normal ranges printed on reports as gospel. Blood chemistries fall either inside or outside the normal range, "and never the twain shall meet." I do the same thing when dealing with tests outside my narrow field of expertise.

Subspecialists, due to undiluted exposure, day in and day out, to patients with a limited set of problems, develop a sort of internal clock: a sense of whether a result is high, low, or normal that is not necessarily tied to precise numbers. I don't mean to imply anything mystical, or that endocrinologists don't use published norms. It's just that we bring a level of familiarity, perhaps wisdom, to understanding where the numbers come from—what they mean physiologically—that adds another dimension to their interpretation.

Is It Always Normal to Be Normal?

Suppose Angela's thyrotropin (TSH) level is 4.5 mU/L, with a normal range on paper of 0.3–5.0 mU/L. It would be true to say "Angela the number" is *statistically* normal. Does that mean "Angela the person" is *physiologically* normal? According to the assumptions behind the standards of care presented last chapter, yes. Doctors don't even consider treatment for low thyroid unless TSH exceeds 5.0 mU/L, right? And some, not even then.

What if Angela also has four of the twelve low-thyroid findings on the Zulewski list? Throw in a family history of thyroid disease. What if she also has a free thyroxine (FT_4) level of 0.8 nanograms per deciliter (ng/dl), where the normal range is 0.7–1.5 ng/dl? Based on her Zulewski score, Angela is clinically borderline low thyroid. Remember, *clinically* refers to the patient's complaints and the physician's five senses. Angela also has a better-than-average risk of developing hypothyroidism because thyroid problems run in her family. Plus, she has a high-normal TSH and a low-normal FT_4. We know TSH goes up as FT_4 goes down. This pattern reeks of abnormality, though the report from the lab labels all the numbers normal.

Does it matter that both the TSH and FT_4 test results fall within a few tenths of a point of being abnormal? I think it does. Should Angela be treated for hypothyroidism? The standards of care say no. I think she should and I can justify that position as long as I consider what the normal range of any blood test really represents.

Shades of Normal

What is normal? My dictionary lists eight definitions, but for our purposes, two will suffice: (1) absence of disease, and (2) a bell-shaped frequency distribution in which 95 percent of all results are within two standard deviations of the average value. The first statement is a physiological definition, the second a statistical one. The latter says, if you take a bunch of healthy volunteers and run Test A on them, the middle 95 percent are "normal." So, Test A's normal range is where 95 percent of results fall when the test is run on people who supposedly don't have the disease Test A looks for.

Two things are worrisome here. First, how do we know those "healthy" volunteers are really healthy? Mild hypothyroidism, we've said, is easy to miss. If so, some normal ranges might be based on data from people who were thyroid deficient but didn't know it. Second, if Test A's normal range reflects 95 percent of healthy people, then by definition the remaining 5 percent of healthy people must have results for Test A falling outside the normal range: 2.5 percent above, another 2.5 percent below.

Some healthy people have abnormal test results, not because of error, but because of statistics. And if that is so, couldn't the opposite be true—unhealthy people have normal tests? Sure, and laboratory medicine experts acknowledge this. That's why they prefer the term *reference range* to *normal range*. They don't want doctors doing what they so often do—equate numbers within the reference range with the absence of disease.

The Individual versus the Population

There is also the important concept of individual reference range. Concentrations of substances in the blood, like thyroid hormone, are tightly regulated, but every person is a little different. Different shaped nose, different personality, different blood chemistry profile. Thus, the fluctuations of FT_4 levels within the same person from one day to the next should be less than the fluctuation of FT_4 between different people. Put another way, if the FT_4 range in 100 average Americans tested on the same day is 0.7–1.5 ng/dl, then the FT_4 range in an individual—we'll call her Rachel—if we drew her blood daily for 100 consecutive days—ouch!—might be 0.8–1.1 ng/dl. Do the same with another healthy woman, Cynthia, and her range might be 1.2–1.4 ng/dl. Both women fall within the population reference range of 0.7–1.5 ng/dl, but their individual reference ranges don't even overlap.

A study in the *Journal of Clinical Endocrinology and Metabolism* did essentially what I described. Thyroid tests were run monthly on sixteen healthy men for a year. Researchers found that the average gap between the highest readings and the lowest readings for an individual was about half as large as the average gap when the numbers for all sixteen men were lumped together. This is an important but confusing point, so allow me to elaborate:

Subject A in the study had twelve readings taken over the course of a year, each of which came out a little different. For example, say that subject A's highest level was 10.0 and his lowest was 7.0. Subject A's gap was 3.0 (10.0 – 7.0 = 3.0). Now, for a second man, subject B: his highest level over the year was 6.0, his lowest was 4.0, with a gap of 2.0 (6.0 – 4.0 = 2.0). The average gap for these two subjects, treated as individuals, is (3.0 + 2.0) ÷ 2 = 2.5. The group average gap though is different. In January, subject A's level was 10.0 and subject B's was 4.0; in February, subject A's level was 7.0 and subject B's was 6.0. I'm not going to extend this example to cover all sixteen men or all twelve months, but just going with what we have so far—the group gap in January is 10.0 – 4.0 = 6.0, in February, 7.0 – 6.0 = 1.0. For these two months, the average gap for the group was 3.5 ([6.0 + 1.0] ÷ 2). So, in this simple example, the average individual gap was 2.5 and the average group gap was 3.5. The numbers vary more in groups (that is, in populations) than in individuals. The authors of this study concluded that "a test result within the laboratory reference limits [the population norm] is not necessarily normal for the individual."

Back to Rachel and Cynthia. Both go to the doctor a year later complaining about fatigue, weight gain, and hair loss. Hypothyroidism is suspected. Both have an FT_4 test done. Rachel's result is 0.7 ng/dl and Cynthia's in 0.9 ng/dl. Both numbers are normal according to the printed reference range of 0.7–1.5 ng/dl, so their doctors decide they don't need treatment. However, Rachel's FT_4 is 0.1 point below her individual reference range established a year earlier; Cynthia's is 0.3 points below hers. Both women are hypothyroid relative to their personal needs. If their TSH levels were tested, they'd probably come out mildly high.

Normal ranges are helpful, but they shouldn't dictate interpretation. I'm proposing nothing radical. I could have quoted a very similar discussion out of my 2161-page endocrinology textbook—a tome representing the very core of mainstream endocrine practice. It's just that busy doctors often forget to take a breath, step back, and question results. Plus, endocrinologists have pounded it into those primary-care doctors that thyroid diagnosis is virtually all about test results. They're doing what they've been taught, but sometimes it's wrong.

Statistically versus Physiologically Normal

We've just shown that an individual with test results within the population's reference range can still be abnormal. Population data is not, therefore, always applicable to the individual. And what if the population reference range isn't even applicable to the population? What if the reference range is wrong? What if the *statistical* normal range does not equal the *physiological* normal range?

A simple example should illustrate this point. There is an epidemic of obesity. In 1999, 61 percent of Americans between the ages of twenty and seventy-four were reported to be overweight or frankly obese. According to the National Institutes of Health (NIH), for a man of my height—five feet, five inches—a healthy (that is, *physiologically normal*) weight is between 114 and 144 pounds. Now, I don't know what the weight range of the middle 95 percent of five-foot, five-inch American men is (fitting the definition of *statistically normal*). But if 61 percent of them are overweight or obese, this weight range won't be between 114 and 144 pounds; I'm guessing it's closer to a range between 130 and 210 pounds, with an average of perhaps 168 pounds. Based on these assumptions, a man of my height who weighs 168 pounds would be statistically normal. But, physiologically, he would be twenty-two pounds heavy, and facing a higher risk of heart disease and diabetes.

The more common a disease is, the less accurate straight statistics become for medical purposes. For a rampant problem like obesity, it's critical to get away from the concept of normal being what is most frequent. Unfortunately, that's the easiest way to go. It's much harder to decide at what weight the risk of problems like heart attack and diabetes starts to climb. But that's what the NIH did when it said 144 pounds was the upper normal weight for men my size.

So it is with TSH. According to the Third National Health and Nutritional Examination Survey (NHANES III), 9.6 million Americans are hypothyroid, which the researchers defined as having a TSH greater than 4.5 mU/L. That means about 5 percent of the total United States population twelve years old or older has low thyroid. Therefore, even without considering the problems surrounding underdiagnosis, hypothyroidism is so common that when interpreting TSH results, a distinction must be made between *statistically* normal (the 0.3–5.0 mU/L range) and *physiologically* normal.

Redefining Normal TSH

Before 1995, I would have had to confess at this point, to indulging in educated speculation. It became evident to me during and after my training that people with TSH levels in the upper half of the reference range tended to feel unwell and seemed to benefit from thyroid hormone pills. And in those already taking pills, it was often inadequate to simply get their TSH somewhere inside that 0.3 mU/L to 5.0 mU/L zone. They felt better with a TSH in the lower half of that range (less than about 2.5 mU/L).

I wasn't the only one noticing this. Treating low-thyroid patients with enough thyroid hormone to get the TSH to low-normal levels was a standard recommendation even back then from experts at places like Harvard and the NIH. Yet, those same professors were saying don't *start* treatment unless the TSH goes above 5.0 mU/L, or maybe 10.0 mU/L. They were confident enough that a high-normal TSH was bad to state that the goal of therapy should be lower, but that didn't translate to a lower threshold for initiating therapy. I have a problem with that, though I do understand it. It hearkens back to "first, do no harm." Doctors have to overcome a lot of inertia before starting a pill, but once a person is on one, the sky's the limit.

So, I was concluding by the mid-1990s that while TSHs in the upper half of the reference range might be statistically normal, they weren't physiologically ideal. It seemed logical to me that mild hypothyroidism, causing slight TSH elevations of 2.5–5.0 mU/L, might be so prevalent that it was skewing the TSH normal range upward. Such TSH levels— still called "normal" today—were normal because they were common, not because they signified health. As it turns out, the National Academy of

Clinical Biochemistry (NACB) said almost exactly the same thing in their recent practice guidelines: "Given the high prevalence of mild . . . hypothyroidism in the general population, it is likely that the current upper limit of the population reference range is skewed by the inclusion of persons with occult thyroid dysfunction."

In 1995, a group of researchers in the United Kingdom published a paper in which they revisited the Whickham Study. The original Whickham Study, from the early 1970s, was a survey of the frequency of thyroid disease in a large free-living population. One of the startling findings of the follow-up report was that people who had a TSH above 2.0 mU/L in the first study had a sharply increased rate of diagnosed hypothyroidism twenty years later. That suggested TSHs above 2.0 mU/L were not entirely normal.

The icing on the cake for me was a paper presented at the 2002 American Thyroid Association meeting in Los Angeles. It reported thyroid test results from more than 17,000 American teenagers and adults done as part of NHANES III. Researchers found the prevalence of thyroid-peroxidase antibodies (TPOAbs) in men was lowest in those with a TSH under 2.0 mU/L. In women, TPOAb tests were least likely to be positive when the TSH was below 1.5 mU/L. In both groups, TPOAb positivity increased proportionally with increasing TSHs above 1.5 mU/L in women or 2.0 mU/L in men. None of the subjects had an abnormal total T_4 level or any known thyroid history. The overall prevalence of positive TPOAbs—which the authors equated with possible undiagnosed hypothyroidism—was 11.2 percent. These researchers, from the University of Southern California, the University of Kansas, and Boston University, drew two conclusions germane to our discussion: (1) undiagnosed hypothyroidism is common in Americans of all ages and ethnicities, and (2) the upper limit of the normal range for serum TSH should be lowered to 2.0 mU/L.

Two point zero is exactly the same value suggested by the follow-up Whickham Study, except in the British paper this new upper limit was suggested by long-term outcomes. Levels of TSH exceeding 2.0 mU/L predicted the eventual diagnosis of unequivocal hypothyroidism. In the American study, TSH levels greater than 2.0 mU/L were associated with thyroid antibodies, markers of incipient hypothyroidism, being found in the blood.

Two studies, two continents, two totally different kinds of data—yet they supported *exactly* the same conclusion. TSH levels greater than 2.0 mU/L aren't normal. Interestingly, this suggested new upper limit for TSH falls quite close to the 2.5 mU/L I've used for years as my own personal upper limit when deciding how to treat my patients.

Low-thyroid management didn't change, however, after the NHANES paper was presented. For one thing, no real-world laboratory I know of is using the new range. It was merely a suggestion, one that I think will eventually be adopted. Of course, the old upper limit of about 5.0 mU/L has been in place for as long as I can remember, yet some guidelines still waffle about treating anything under 10.0 mU/L. Nothing will change quickly, but this new data does bolster those of us who think most TSHs above 4.0–5.0 mU/L should be treated and leads me to believe we should at least consider therapy when TSHs exceed 2.0 mU/L.

In fairness to mainstream academia, they are—finally—affording this issue an open debate. Two articles in major endocrinology journals in late 2005 advocated lowering treatment thresholds for TSH testing. One made the bold (for a peer-reviewed paper) statement that people with TSHs greater than 3.0 mU/L should get treatment and that therapy should be considered when the test exceeds 2.5 mU/L. An opposing position was also published, reiterating the questionable benefits of treating any TSH less than 10.0 mU/L.

Some months before those articles appeared, I had the lucky opportunity to discuss my position on treating TSHs greater than 2.0 mU/L with one of the authors of the opposition article. Not surprisingly—in retrospect, now that I've read his paper—he emphatically disagreed with me. His reasoning, in so many words, was that TSH tests run in laboratories in Podunk, U.S.A., couldn't be trusted enough to be accurate. He might have a point, but it's interesting and illuminating, I think, how the academic elite disparages doctors' ability to conduct themselves out in the real world. More on that later.

Here is a situation where hardcore reformists and I agree. Blood testing gets it wrong. Yet, we've just done something the reformist literature, in my experience, doesn't—we've said that TSH testing misses some people with hypothyroidism, and we've shown why and suggested corrective action. They just say blood tests don't work, so don't do them. That's the wrong conclusion to draw.

Let's look back at Cynthia. She had a few symptoms and a low-normal FT_4 of 0.9 ng/dl. Let's say her TSH was 3.3 mU/L with our usual normal range of 0.3–5.0 mU/L. Nine out of ten times she'll be told her tests are normal, so it can't be her thyroid. But if she were to see me for a second opinion, I would tell her that her thyroid levels are mildly low and treatment is an option. Those conclusions would be based on the TSH exceeding 2.0 mU/L, plus the somewhat low FT_4, plus her symptoms.

That's not the only possible correct course. Lifelong drug therapy, after all, isn't to be taken lightly. Repeating Cynthia's tests in three months would be reasonable, possibly adding a TPOAb to assess the risk of future worsening of the condition. On the other hand, I have treated many patients right away in this situation. I might write her a prescription that day if she simply wanted me to or if she had severe symptoms such as a goiter, high cholesterol, depression, or if she had numerous borderline TSH results in the past, suggesting the problem isn't likely to just vanish. Mine is an aggressive approach, however. You might not easily find a doctor willing to do the same.

HOW MUCH HYPOTHYROIDISM IS MISSED?

I opened this book by saying that some reformists condemn blood testing because it misses a lot of hypothyroidism, and I've bolstered that position with both speculation and fact. But how many low-thyroid sufferers are being missed?

Particularly compelling in this regard is a 2002 analysis of the U.S. Centers for Disease Control's NHANES III databank, which showed the overall prevalence of hypothyroidism (defined by them as a TSH greater than 4.5 mU/L) in the United States to be 4.6 percent of the population. That figure is almost four times higher than the most generous estimates cited by earlier work.

Let's crunch some numbers. The above-mentioned analysis suggested that 9.6 million Americans were biochemically hypothyroid during the NHANES III study period (1988–1994). Of those, 1.6 million knew they had a problem but weren't getting treatment or weren't on enough medication. The remaining 8 million were *undiagnosed*—that is, an estimated 8 million people with low thyroid in the United States were completely missed by the healthcare system. In the study, 10.4 million Americans self-reported having thyroid disease. That figure wasn't broken down as to type of thyroid problem (high levels, low levels, goiters, nodules), but using other data, I can guess that 8.2 million of them were probably hypothyroid. That's consistent with the oft-quoted figure of 8–12 million Americans taking thyroid hormone pills.

So, about 8.2 million Americans know they have hypothyroidism and an additional 8 million are hypothyroid and don't know it. That means close to half of Americans with true hypothyroidism, defined as a TSH greater than 4.5 mU/L, are being missed. Half. And that doesn't even get into patients with hypothyroidism whose TSHs don't go up that high, including those with central hypothyroidism or very mild thyroid failure. The point is, mainstream research clearly supports the notion that hypothyroidism is underdiagnosed.

At this juncture, though, I submit that a great many low-thyroid patients *are* identified, using reference ranges and standards of practice recognized by everybody walking out of medical school. Cases in point— the 8.2 million self-reported hypothyroid patients documented by NHANES III and the 8–12 million said to take thyroid pills every day. Family practitioners, internists, gynecologists, and thousands of endocrinologists do fine diagnosing and treating many people every day. So throwing out the tests that got us this far would be absurd. The situation is bad enough *with* these tools, I shudder to think where we'd be *without* them.

The matter for debate is: How many are we missing? Are we picking up a majority or a minority of the actual cases? I don't know. NHANES III suggests we neglect half of those with TSHs above 4.5 mU/L. How many more do we add for central and mild primary hypothyroidism in which TSHs don't exceed 4.5 mU/L? We could be looking at a 60 to 70 percent underdiagnosis rate.

WHAT'S THE SOLUTION?

So, yes, we do miss a lot. But a significant portion of those cases could be found using the same tools available today, provided doctors change two things about the way they interpret thyroid function tests:

1. Move the normal range of TSH down to 2.0 or 2.5 mU/L.

2. Recognize that a normal FT_4 on paper does not always mean the individual's thyroid-hormone needs are being met.

The numbers aren't necessarily faulty—what we do with them is. My proposed guidelines for deciphering thyroid blood tests are as follows:

1. Most people with TSHs greater than 5.0 mU/L should be called hypothyroid and treated, especially if multiple checks exceed 5.0 mU/L for months or years (and provided rare instances where a high TSH is accompanied by high thyroid levels are ruled out).

2. Most people with TSHs of 2.0–5.0 mU/L are probably mildly hypothyroid and treatment should be considered, especially in those with:

   • Multiple clinical findings or a single one that is especially severe.

   • Family history of thyroid disease.

   • Coexistence of any of the following: infertility, menstrual disorders, dyslipidemia, psychiatric disease (especially depression), goiter, thyroid nodule(s), positive TPOAb test, or pregnancy.

3. A normal result on any T_4 or T_3 test precludes *none* of the above.

4. Most people with TSH levels less than 2.0 mU/L are not hypothyroid and do not require treatment. (Exceptions to this rule will be the subject of the next two chapters.)

CHAPTER 5

ATYPICAL HYPOTHYROIDISM: CENTRAL DEFECTS

In the last chapter, we listed three ways a true low-thyroid condition might be missed:

- The doctor is faulty.

- The standard of care is faulty.

- The tests are faulty.

We then detailed common mistakes doctors make using thyroid tests and discussed systemic errors in how these studies have come to be interpreted. These problems encompass the first two items on our list and are correctable with research and training. They are behavioral issues, and behaviors can be changed. Now, we'll attack the technology—the failure of current biochemical testing to detect subtle or esoteric ("atypical") forms of hypothyroidism. That is, in the best of hands, those of the most progressively open-minded of practitioners, there are still true low-thyroid patients that blood tests don't identify.

MURPHY'S LAW OF THE THYROID

Murphy's Law is not a scientific law. It doesn't carry the same weight as one of Newton's laws of thermodynamics, but it is common sense. If something can go wrong, it will go wrong. It might go wrong half the time, or one in a hundred times, or one in a million times, but at some point everything breaks. Why should Murphy's Law be any less applicable to medicine than to the rest of human experience? Some medical problems are common and some are exceedingly rare. Some are so minor as to be unrecognizable and some are so serious as to cause death in the womb. But it doesn't make sense to me that there could be any process in human physiology that never derails.

We have been focusing largely on the hypothalamic-pituitary-thyroid (HPT) axis. The debate over exactly what TSH level to call "normal" affects doctors' ability to diagnose defects in the thyroid gland and, to a lesser degree, in the brain and pituitary gland. However, what about failure of peripheral conversion of T_4 to T_3 in remote reaches of the body? What about problems with thyroid hormone receptors at the core of individual cells? What about . . . ? You see my point.

Doctors focus on *primary* hypothyroidism—disease contained within the thyroid gland. Exceptions, while acknowledged, are assumed to be rare. But what if they aren't rare? Even if they are, physicians are still obligated to recognize and manage uncommon problems. In this chapter and the next, I will spotlight the limits of our current comprehension of thyroid system physiology and the deficiencies of laboratory science with respect to it.

Starting from the top, there are nine points where something theoretically could go awry within the thyroid system, and a tenth point I feel compelled to add:

1. Thyrotropin-releasing hormone (TRH) production and release by the brain

2. Thyrotropin (TSH, thyroid-stimulating hormone) production and release by the pituitary gland

3. Thyroxine (T_4) and triiodothyronine (T_3) production and release by the thyroid gland

4. Binding and release of T_4 and T_3 by transport proteins

5. Entry of T_4 and T_3 into cells all over the body, including in the brain and pituitary

6. Conversion of T_4 to T_3 by deiodinases all over the body, including in the brain and pituitary

7. Entry of T_3 into the nuclei of cells all over the body, including in the brain and pituitary

8. Binding of T_3 to the thyroid hormone receptor attached to each cell's DNA

9. Activation of the thyroid hormone receptor

10. Balancing central and peripheral thyroid hormone actions

Each level of this system depends on the other levels. Regulation of hypothalamic (brain) synthesis and secretion of TRH (point 1), for example, is modulated by peripheral conversion of T_4 to T_3 in the hypothalamus (point 6). I repeated the phrase "all over the body, including in the brain and pituitary" to emphasize that thyroid hormone actions in these "elite" tissues may or may not match what's going on in the rest of the body. What if Susan's brain and pituitary—which directly impact her HPT axis, controlling how much thyroid hormone the rest of her body gets—aren't in sync with the rest of Susan? Trouble, that's what—a thyroid system out of balance. This brings up the tenth point in the process—balancing central and peripheral actions.

Central refers to the brain and pituitary (points 1 and 2), everything in the thyroid system above the thyroid gland. *Peripheral* refers to the thyroid gland and everything below it (points 3 to 9). In this chapter and the next, we will discuss things that might go wrong at each of these levels.

POINTS 1 AND 2—BRAIN AND PITUITARY PROBLEMS

Trauma and disease involving the pituitary gland, hypothalamus, and other areas of the brain can disrupt TRH and TSH production. This causes central hypothyroidism, in which TSH fails to increase adequately in the face of thyroid hormone deficiency.

Too frequently, doctors don't entertain the possibility of central hypothyroidism when evaluating their patients. Every time a TSH test is used alone to check a patient for low-thyroid, central hypothyroidism is being automatically dismissed. If TSH is normal, doctors think: it can't be thyroid. Oh, but it can. If they were to check a free thyroxine (FT_4) level, and it turned out to be low despite that normal TSH, the central defect might be exposed. Strictly speaking, then, failure to diagnose central hypothyroidism is often a doctor failure, not a technology failure. But since it is a situation where the commonplace rules for interpreting TSH levels don't apply, I'm lumping it here under the umbrella of atypical hypothyroidism.

No doctor, certainly no endocrinologist, should often miss *severe* central hypothyroidism: the patient has symptoms, perhaps a history of head trauma or pituitary tumor, her TSH is normal or low, and her FT_4 is low. Based on the evidence, a correct diagnosis should be made—it might not be, but I'm an optimist. However, what about mild to moderate, as opposed to severe, central hypothyroidism? Many people with mild primary hypothyroidism show normal FT_4 and FT_3 levels. Remember, they can be below the individual's normal range and still be normal relative to the population according to the laboratory report. The same principle holds true for central hypothyroidism, meaning that there are cases of central hypothyroidism in which TSH is normal or low and the FT_4 is normal—a very hard diagnosis to make, especially on tests alone.

Recall Cynthia with the individual FT_4 normal range of 1.2–1.4 nanograms per deciliter (ng/dl). Let's say she once suffered a concussion in a traffic accident, a possible cause of central hypothyroidism. She goes to her doctor complaining of fatigue, hair loss, and depression. He checks TSH and FT_4. The TSH is 1.5 milliunits per liter (mU/L) and the FT_4 is 0.9 ng/dl, both values normal according to the report. They're also both normal based on my own criteria detailed at the end of the last chapter. Cynthia is not biochemically hypothyroid even by this author's standards. But she does have chronic fatigue, her hair is falling out, and she's depressed. Clinically, there is reason to suspect low thyroid and reason to suspect hypothalamic or pituitary damage (i.e., that head injury).

How can her doctor confirm that she actually has mild central hypothyroidism that needs treatment? The best way is the TRH-stimulation test described earlier, in which we try to spark TSH production from the pituitary and measure its response. If we are correct about central hypothyroidism, her doctor should find a blunting or delay in the rise of TSH. Unfortunately, her doctor can't do that test because Thyrel (TRH) is off the market. Unless and until it comes back, the only way to manage this patient correctly is to *suspect* low thyroid, *ignore* her normal blood tests, and give thyroid hormone pills anyway.

By the way, the astute reader might be saying: "Obviously she's hypothyroid, since her actual FT_4 of 0.9 ng/dl was below her individual normal range of 1.2–1.4." Yes, but I gave you that information for clarity. Everyone has an individual reference range, but doctors have no practical way of knowing what it is.

Cynthia's story is a plausible scenario meshing precisely with the reformist thesis that some people with perfect thyroid tests nevertheless may have true hypothyroidism. Even the hoped for return of Thyrel would not fix that situation. Physicians will still need to look beyond the normal blood tests, register the clinical abnormalities, and think about the need for TRH testing, which never has been an everyday test for most doctors.

Occult Central Hypothyroidism (OCH)

Besides obvious disease or trauma involving the head, which most doctors *should* take into account when interpreting thyroid blood tests, there are a number of obscure causes of low TSH release that might be missed even by a good endocrinologist—hence, my coining of the term *occult central hypothyroidism* (OCH).

Hypothalamic-pituitary-thyroid axis interference of the type that might create OCH can be seen in starvation states, including the condition anorexia nervosa, and possibly in massive obesity (largely speculation on my part, based on observation; however, I've seen no published studies supporting an obesity–HPT axis connection). Certain drugs—dopamine, used only in the critically ill, the anti-epileptic phenytoin, and the widely prescribed antidiabetic drug metformin—can block HPT axis function. And, there are cases where the pituitary makes so-called bio-inactive TSH, a defective hormone that doesn't adequately stimulate the thyroid gland.

However, I think that most OCH is caused by HPT-axis suppression from either adrenal steroid excess or, paradoxically, past hyperthyroid (high-thyroid) conditions. Because these factors are of such importance in the creation of the thyroid paradox, I will describe each in detail below.

Post-Hyperthyroid OCH

*Hypo*thyroidism is the medical term for low thyroid. *Hyper*thyroidism means high thyroid, also a relatively common disorder in women (and some men) of all ages. Ironically, I suspect past hyperthyroidism to be one of the most common causes of occult central hypothyroidism. It is well known that most hyperthyroid patients will, for one reason or another, end up being hypothyroid. Mostly this is because proper therapy of a high-thyroid state often renders the person permanently hypothyroid, either from surgical removal of, or radiation damage to, the thyroid gland. The need usually arises, therefore, for patients to begin taking thyroid hormone pills soon after such treatment. This is *primary* hypothyroidism resulting from thyroid destruction, a side effect of high-thyroid therapy.

Central hypothyroidism, on the other hand, occurs as a lingering consequence of the high-thyroid condition itself—not a side effect of treatment, but a side effect of the disease. When thyroxine (T_4) rises in hyperthyroidism, thyrotropin (TSH) declines. This is the normal negative feedback. By the time thyroid levels are high enough to require treatment, TSH production has usually fallen to nothing, as has thyrotropin-releasing hormone (TRH) production from the hypothalamus. In other words, hyperthyroidism suppresses hypothalamic-pituitary-thyroid axis function. If there is an abundance of thyroid hormone, the body has no reason to make more. Everything related to TRH and TSH production goes on hiatus: the body's machinery gets dismantled and put away; the factory workers are laid off.

If suppression of the HPT axis by hyperthyroidism is short-lived, no problem. Normal function kicks back in soon after the high-thyroid state is corrected. After thyroid levels fall, TRH rises, followed by TSH. On the other hand, if inhibition of the central part of the system has been prolonged, a "use it or lose it" phenomenon happens, like muscles wasting in a bedridden patient. The HPT axis doesn't reawaken as readily, and TSH levels don't climb as T_4 levels fall.

Now, when forced back to work, shriveled muscles eventually recover. So it is with the TRH-secreting cells of the brain and the TSH-secreting cells of the pituitary. Eventually, the hypothyroid state will force those cells back to work. But what if they aren't forced? You see, primary hypothyroidism following treatment for hyperthyroidism is fully expected, even desired. Doctors watch for it. At the first sign of low-thyroid hormone levels, the conscientious physician leaps to the rescue, giving thyroid pills to spare the patient as much discomfort as possible. I did this countless times myself—before learning better. And this I learned, by the way, through experience, not at all from a textbook, journal article, or lecture.

There are two problems with immediately correcting post-treatment primary hypothyroidism. First, if thyroid hormone pills were withheld until after the HPT axis awakened, perhaps TSH would stimulate T_4 and T_3 production from whatever remained of the thyroid, and lifelong pills might be avoided. That *could* happen but probably won't in most cases, so that scenario is not my biggest concern.

What does worry me is something we've already talked about: doctors focus almost exclusively on TSH levels when diagnosing hypothyroidism and when regulating dosages of thyroid pills. In the post-hyperthyroid patient, however, thyroid hormone replacement therapy removes the stimulus for the pituitary to ever make TSH again. If all or most of the body's thyroid requirements are met by a pill, why waste resources making TSH to tell the thyroid to make something that isn't needed?

Physiologically that's okay—you and I don't need TSH. The problem is when an unsuspecting doctor stumbles along and (as almost all do) uses TSH testing in trying to determine the correct thyroid hormone dose. If the HPT axis never recovered from its slumber, the TSH will forever be lower than it should be for any given T_4 level. The thyroid's gauge is broken. And since the situation is analogous to a car's gas gauge being stuck on "F," the patient may be given insufficient thyroid hormone by her doctor—similar to a car not getting a fill-up from its owner, because of the erroneous instrument, despite a nearly empty tank.

To recap, the patient recently treated for high thyroid has two low-thyroid problems:

- Primary hypothyroidism as a side effect of treatment (common knowledge)

- Central hypothyroidism as a lingering effect of the hyperthyroidism (not common knowledge)

Jessica's Fall into Thyroid Purgatory

Jessica, with a free thyroxine (FT_4) individual normal range of 1.4–1.7 ng/dl, has Graves' disease. This condition is the most common internal cause of hyperthyroidism. Radioactive iodine is prescribed to destroy her out-of-control thyroid. Before treatment, her FT_4 is high at 3.5 ng/dl and her TSH is very low at less than 0.01 mU/L. As expected, two months later, her FT_4 becomes low at 0.4 ng/dl, but her TSH is still less than 0.01 mU/L.

Her doctor knows that TSH often remains low *for a short time* after treatment (delayed recovery of the HPT axis). She even recognizes that eventual HPT axis recovery may raise FT_4 levels. "Let's wait and see," she tells Jessica, hoping to avoid ordering lifelong thyroid hormone therapy. A month passes and Jessica complains bitterly of low-thyroid symptoms. Her FT_4 is even lower at 0.2 ng/dl and her TSH is now high at 8.5 mU/L.

Time to get down to work. Jessica has symptoms, and her FT_4 is still falling despite resumption of TSH production. In fact, her TSH is clearly high. Jessica's doctor thinks her patient is permanently hypothyroid and she's probably right. The drug Synthroid is prescribed at the moderate dose of 100 micrograms (mcg) per day. So far, so good.

Eight weeks later, Jessica feels better, though some symptoms remain. Her TSH is 0.12 mU/L. Anything under 0.3 mU/L in a patient taking thyroid pills generally triggers a lowering of the dose. The doctor didn't order an FT_4 test this time—it wasn't needed, she reasoned, since the TSH was high last time. Jessica's HPT axis has recovered. TSH is once again the be-all and end-all indicator of thyroid status.

"What about my symptoms?" Jessica is reassured they will improve with time—"or maybe they're not caused by your thyroid at all." But since her TSH is low, her Synthroid dose is lowered to 88 mcg per day. Jessica returns six weeks later feeling worse, but on a happier note the TSH is normal, a pristine 1.8 ng/dl. Jessica is told her thyroid medicine is well regulated and she should return in six months. "Wait, wait," she pleads, "I still feel horrible."

A conscientious search for other problems finds nothing. Jessica is told to give it more time. It can take months to recover from the ravages of hyperthyroidism. Maybe she needs more exercise, or more rest, or to cut her hours at work, or to learn to handle stress better. At Jessica's insistence, her doctor orders an FT_4 test just to be sure. It's 1.2 ng/dl, which is well within the lab's reference range. Jessica is told it can't be her thyroid.

And so begins her descent into purgatory, thoroughly ensnared in the thyroid paradox. She is underdosed, but can't convince a doctor of it. Or if she can, the low TSH resulting from each attempt to up her medication prompts the doctor to drop it back down.

Where was the misstep? Obviously, the FT_4 of 1.2 ng/dl, however normal on paper, is below Jessica's personal normal range of 1.4–1.7 ng/dl. Unfortunately, as we've said, no doctor has a way to know that, short of numerous trial-and-error adjustments with meticulous attention to signs and symptoms—something insurance companies would become apoplectic over and modern physicians aren't taught to do. Even if they were, it would be a long, frustrating, impractical process.

Was there any other clue that could have prevented this misadventure? Rewind to the office visit when Jessica was first prescribed Synthroid. Her FT_4 was very low at 0.2 ng/dl and her TSH was mildly high at 8.5 mU/L. The appropriate TSH to accompany an FT_4 level that low is more like 30 or 50 or 100, perhaps 200 mU/L! Her TSH of 8.5 mU/L was high, but less so than it should have been. Her HPT axis had only partly recovered from the effects of hyperthyroidism, and further recovery stopped once she started taking thyroid pills. From that point forward, Jessica's TSH ran lower than it should have, and it probably will continue to do so for the rest of her life, a pattern which will suggest her thyroid levels are higher than they are. Jessica's thyroid gauge is stuck on "F."

There are two ways to fix this, assuming anybody ever realizes it's happening. Stop or greatly lower her dose long enough to drive the TSH really high, forcing recovery of the HPT axis. That could take weeks, months, or a year. The whole time she'll be suffering severe symptoms. The alternative is to simply ignore the TSH and adjust therapy based on symptoms and other blood tests, namely FT_4, and perhaps FT_3 levels.

What could have prevented this problem? In a low-thyroid patient recently treated for hyperthyroidism, I begin thyroid hormone at a low dose, a quarter to a half what I think is really needed. This takes the edge off symptoms without blocking HPT axis recovery. Once the TSH rises convincingly, I adjust the dose upward. And I explain to patients what I'm doing; otherwise they're liable to decide the low dose isn't working and they might not come back—or at the very least they'll go through weeks of unnecessary frustration.

I call this problem *post-hyperthyroid central hypothyroidism* (PHCH), and it receives remarkably little attention in textbooks and medical training. When it does, it's presented as a temporary aberration. Ideally it is, but the well-meaning doctor can make it permanent. Frankly, I don't think I've ever read or heard an expert recommend altering thyroid hormone replacement doses to prevent long-term PHCH, or mention that PHCH could ever last more than a few weeks or months after hyperthyroid therapy. At least not until I talked to a renowned Mayo Clinic thyroidologist in the hall at the 2004 Endocrine Society meeting in New Orleans. I proposed this whole notion to him. He shrugged and said, "Oh, yes, of course."

I think PHCH is widespread, probably the leading cause of missed (or inadequately treated) hypothyroidism after surgical or radioactive-iodine treatment for thyroid excess. I think it's especially common after surgery. Post-operative patients become thyroid deficient essentially instantly, and thyroid pills get started while they're still in the hospital. (I'm only talking here about surgery to cure hyperthyroidism. Most people having thyroid surgery can start pills right away with no problem.) At least with slower-acting radioactive iodine, hypothyroidism takes weeks or months to develop, allowing time for some HPT axis recovery. Another cause of PHCH is HPT-axis suppression from thyroid pills. This problem might result from past overdoses or from TSH levels that have been deliberately rendered low as a treatment for thyroid cancer, goiters, or benign nodules.

PHCH exists, although I'm speculating on how common it is. There is precedent in other hormone systems, though, to support the idea of PHCH being a significant problem. It is common knowledge, for instance, that up to a year may be required for the hypothalamus and pituitary glands to resume proper regulation of the adrenal glands after a period of adrenal hormone excess. And I've seen a number of athletes rendered permanently incapable of making testosterone or sperm by anabolic steroids. Why so little attention has been paid to the analogous situation in the thyroid system boggles me. The organ that gets no respect.

Steroid-Induced OCH

Overload of another group of hormones might also cause occult central hypothyroidism. Glucocorticoids are a life-sustaining type of steroid hormone made by the adrenal glands. The major glucocorticoid is cortisol. Small amounts are produced daily, but in times of stress, such as after trauma or during severe illness or major surgery, lots of cortisol gets pumped into the bloodstream to steel the body against whatever has befallen it. Cortisol increases blood pressure and glucose levels and generally diverts resources away from protein production and immune function, all for the purpose of maintaining blood, oxygen, and fuel flow to the brain in an emergency. Those are all good things, provided the crisis resolves quickly. But exposing the body to even slightly high cortisol levels for long periods can be devastating, even fatal.

The collection of effects inflicted by excess glucocorticoids is called Cushing's syndrome. This condition can be caused by tumors (usually of the pituitary gland or lungs) that stimulate the adrenals or by direct oversecretion from an adrenal tumor. Glucocorticoids taken in pill form—common examples are hydrocortisone (Cortef), cortisone, prednisone, methylprednisolone (Medrol), and dexamethasone (Decadron)—treat a variety of diseases, with Cushing's syndrome occurring as a dangerous common side effect.

Excess cortisol or cortisol-like steroids blunt thyrotropin (TSH) production and block peripheral conversion of inactive thyroxine (T_4) to active triiodothyronine (T_3). Theoretically, then, Cushing's syndrome could cause inadequate stimulation of the thyroid—that is, central hypothyroidism—and poor activation of T_4 to its more potent cousin T_3. A one-two punch to the thyroid system. And without a reliable rise in TSH, neither problem would be easily detected.

Fortunately, severe Cushing's syndrome is rare, except in those taking glucocorticoids as drugs. They, at least, are readily identifiable, except that there is no general recognition that occult low thyroid might be among the risks of steroid therapy. That's not the worst of it. Mild thyroid deficiency, we've said, is often missed and there's every reason to believe mild cortisol excess is too. But even that isn't my greatest worry.

Before continuing, I should emphasize that, while mainstream research acknowledges an influence of glucocorticoids on certain functions within the thyroid system, it has also concluded that Cushing's syndrome does not cause frank hypothyroidism. The explanation given is that TSH production escapes the inhibitory effects of steroids after long exposure.

My concerns are not allayed. If some mild or unusual forms of hypothyroidism are often overlooked, how can we be certain about the papers saying Cushing's syndrome doesn't cause hypothyroidism? Was there no hypothyroidism or no hypothyroidism *detected*? A textbook chapter states: "Cushing's syndrome [patients] have serum free-T_4 concentrations within the normal range." What of it? A lot of people I treat for low thyroid have normal FT_4 levels. FT_4 is an insensitive test, and a normal result does not rule out hypothyroidism.

Even if I'm off base about steroids and the HPT axis, steroidal inhibition of T_4 to T_3 conversion (which is undisputed) could seriously muck up the works all by itself. And what about low-grade, off-and-on, elevations of cortisol? That's a different animal from the constant high levels experienced by most Cushing's syndrome patients. The published findings might not apply.

To illustrate, say that one hour (I'm making these numbers up) of ceaseless steroid bombardment is sufficient to get the HPT axis to ignore glucocorticoid inhibition and resume making TRH, TSH, and thyroid hormone. Suppose, then, that Joyce's HPT axis is exposed to thirty minutes of high cortisol, ten times per day, every day—while getting herself ready for work and the kids ready for school, then again with a tough project at work, then getting away from work early to take a kid to the dentist, and so forth. That's a lot of glucocorticoid, but the faucet is never left on long enough to train the HPT axis to ignore it. Might *that* result in central hypothyroidism, even if full-blown Cushing's syndrome doesn't? I don't know the answer and I doubt anybody does. I'm not sure anybody who counts is even asking the question.

Stress, Depression, and Steroids

Both emotional stress and depression trigger secretion of corticotropin-releasing hormone (CRH) from the brain. CRH is to the adrenals what TRII is to the thyroid: it tells the pituitary gland to tell the adrenals to make cortisol. Thus, stress and depression indirectly increase cortisol production. We've said cortisol blocks T_4 to T_3 conversion and possibly TSH synthesis. CRH also causes the body to make somatostatin, which interferes with TRH production. So, one way or another, stress or depression cause the adrenal system to disrupt the thyroid system. Specifically, stress and depression may cause occult central hypothyroidism, and by interfering with peripheral conversion, a form of thyroid hormone resistance (to be discussed in Chapter 6).

Stress may be killing your thyroid. And not just your thyroid—stress-induced cortisol excess inhibits growth hormone and testosterone production as well. These combined hormonal deficiencies may lead to obesity and an increased risk for diabetes, heart attack, and stroke.

Respected mainstream periodicals and textbooks document the facts presented above. Unfortunately, there is little recognition by average mainstream practitioners of these processes actually affecting patients. What about thyroidologists? Surely they see psychologically mediated cortisol release as a potentially significant problem, don't they?

One afternoon at a meeting in Philadelphia, I participated in a discussion led by a well-known thyroidologist. An audience member (not me) asked: "What about TSH suppression due to depression?"

"That doesn't occur," the speaker shot back. "Anyone seen that or thinks that happens?" No one argued. Later, the subject of central hypothyroidism came up and I asked: "What about depression-induced cortisol excess suppressing the HPT axis and creating central hypothyroidism?"

"That doesn't happen clinically," I was told, and the professor turned away curtly. I found myself wondering: What are they afraid of? What is wrong with open-mindedness and a free exchange of ideas, essentials of the most rigid science?

The meeting broke up and I approached the first questioner. We agreed that we both commonly saw what we perceived to be depression-induced TSH suppression. "CRH is king," he stated. "I'm surprised he didn't know that." Didn't know or was unwilling to even speculate that things as ubiquitous as depression and anxiety could disrupt the TSH/T_4 relationship and lessen the power of, and our confidence in, routine thyroid tests? Any expert will preach that the savvy endocrinologist should be alert for *rare* situations where TSH and T_4 don't tell the full story. It's far different to allow that this state of affairs might be commonplace.

Two days later, still in Philadelphia, I went to another session led by a bright young professor whose name was unfamiliar to me. I took that as a sign he might not be an ivory tower-dwelling giant of close-mindedness. He was in the process of listing things other than hyperthyroidism that might decrease TSH. I asked my question again, "In your experience, does depression and/or anxiety lower TSH?"

"Rather than tell you my experience," he replied benignly, "let me tell you the literature (that is, the research)." He proceeded to describe acutely psychotic patients admitted to mental hospitals, who had low TSHs. Their TSH levels went back to normal within days of antipsychotic treatment. Next question. . . . I wasn't asking about delusional people in need of commitment. My concern is the overstressed, mildly depressed "soccer moms" out there slogging through overly hectic days.

Besides, what's wrong with presenting his experience? Last time I checked, the first step in the scientific method was to cast a hypothesis onto the water to be proved or refuted. Yet, the endocrine establishment seems downright fearful of any hypothesizing "outside the lines" in this area.

A year later, at another meeting, another professor from another world-class medical school was pontificating about the new TSH normal range we covered earlier. Paraphrasing, he said: "It's nice for us endocrinologists to talk about, but we don't want this to get out around the country." I was flabbergasted by what amounted to a conspiracy of silence. He was talking about mild *primary* hypothyroidism, not *central* hypothyroidism as we are in this chapter, but the basic issue is the same. "They" don't want doctors in routine practice looking at a normal or mildly abnormal TSH level with any suspicion. "They" think they're protecting patients from unnecessary treatment. Maybe they are, but they're also saying that your family physician can't be trusted with the latest advances in thyroid science. Perhaps rank-and-file doctors would be better doctors if academics stopped keeping secrets and let them have more say about what's best for their own patients.

The Stress-Steroid-Thyroid Connection

My hypothesis is that the chronically overstressed, mildly depressed soccer mom experiences a psychiatrically generated off-and-on elevation of CRH, resulting in low-grade intermittent cortisol excess, which suppresses the HPT axis and other areas of the thyroid system, and possibly other metabolism-regulating hormone systems. The end result is weight gain and fatigue. This scenario is largely consistent with what I was told about the acutely psychotic patient: a psychiatric disturbance results in decreased TSH, then drug treatment eradicates the disturbance and everything goes back to normal? Except the soccer mom might not get treatment. She simply perseveres: keeps dealing with kids, husband, work, meals, finances, plumber, softball practice, dance lessons, and so on. Antidepressant or antianxiety pills, if she gets them, may or may not solve the problem. If the cause of her depression or anxiety is life stress, part of the treatment has to be life change. That's my hypothesis.

My experience, on the other hand, is that I commonly see young women with mildly low TSH levels, whose doctors have referred them because they suspect hyperthyroidism. Generally, high-thyroid sufferers have a TSH level that is too low to measure. So, when I get one that's only a little low, I rule out hyperthyroidism and start trying to figure out what, if anything, *is* wrong. It might be what I call "soccer mom syndrome": stress begets high cortisol, which begets low TSH. I inquire about anxiety, depression, and stress. Frequently, one or more of the answers are yes, at which point I typically reassure her and her doctor that she is not hyper-thyroid. The low TSH is an endocrinologically inconsequential result of psychosocial issues.

But are the results inconsequential or are these folks truly deficient in thyroid hormone? If so, is a thyroid hormone pill the answer? If the underlying cause is lifestyle, no pill will fix that totally. Similarly, no medical treatment will completely arrest emphysema in a person who's still smoking, but doctors do treat emphysema in smokers. Should they give thyroid hormone treatment to soccer moms? There's nothing approaching a standard of care on this issue. If there is, it is not to treat, because low TSHs are taken to suggest high rather than low thyroid levels—unless the person has central hypothyroidism, which the mainstream says is rare.

How rare? Central hypothyroidism is said to occur in about five of every 100,000 people. Compare this to the NHANES III evidence that five of every 100 people have primary hypothyroidism. Mainstream opinion, therefore, says that for every 1,000 people with primary hypothyroidism, only one person has central hypothyroidism. But if our assertions about the frequency of missed primary hypothyroidism are anywhere close to accurate, how many cases of central thyroid deficiency—a harder diagnosis to make—must we be missing? Possibly a lot. I think central hypothyroidism might be very common. I also fear the number of sufferers might be growing in proportion to the degree of stress and lack of downtime in our hectic, cell-phone/instant-messaging/voice-mail/e-mail-connected, 24/7 lives.

Links between body and mind, which have been long suspected, are only now being explained scientifically. Until this research finds its way into the clinic in the form of practical, peer-reviewed recommendations, we're stuck taking a common sense, seat-of-the-pants approach. We can ignore the possibility of stress-induced thyroid dysfunction or we can try to do something about it. If we choose the latter, do we give pills to counter the effects of stress or do we get rid of the stress? There's probably a role for both. Personal responsibility is crucial, but doctors have a responsibility too—to help, or at least do no harm. How best to fulfill that responsibility, in this instance, remains a question for debate.

CHAPTER 6

ATYPICAL HYPOTHYROIDISM: PERIPHERAL DEFECTS

In this chapter, we will continue down the list of ways the thyroid train might jump the rails, which we began in Chapter 5. We have covered the top (central) part of the system—the brain and the pituitary gland. Now, we'll hit points south.

POINT 3—MAKING AND SECRETING T_4 AND T_3

We will skip this point since most of the book deals with it. Defects here, by the way, are not atypical. They comprise all cases of *typical* primary hypothyroidism.

POINT 4—TRANSPORT PROTEINS

I am aware of no one suffering a clinically relevant problem due to a breakdown of thyroxine-binding globulin (TBG) or other proteins that carry thyroid hormone in the bloodstream. There are genetic disorders of thyroid hormone transport, none of which is thought to alter the overall function of the system. One reference states: "It is clear that no one of the proteins is required for good health." The basis for these conclusions is the observation that free thyroxine (FT_4) levels don't change when transport protein function is abnormal. In other words, the validity of the mainstream position requires us to assume that serum FT_4 levels accurately reflect tissue thyroxine (T_4) and triiodothyronine (T_3) status. That is, assume the truth of the free hormone hypothesis, which argues that only thyroid hormone free in the serum, not thyroid hormone stuck to proteins, can exert effects on the body.

I'm not convinced we can make that assumption. There is evidence, for example, that transport proteins might, in a very deliberate way, release bound thyroid hormone deep within specific organs and tissues, targeting the cellular uptake of thyroid hormone (see point 5) to the neediest sites. Thus, FT_4 measured in a blood sample may have little to do with FT_4 in a capillary deep inside, say, the quadriceps muscle. Furthermore, certain cells are thought to have surface receptors that bind TBG or other transport proteins, possibly for the purpose of facilitating entry of thyroid hormone into the cell.

Two things are clear: the whole story hasn't been written on thyroid serum transport proteins, and whatever their role, it is probably more complicated and more important than is generally acknowledged by experts or recognized by most doctors. Could the woman with low-thyroid symptoms but normal laboratory tests have a defect in the serum transport of thyroid hormone? Sure, we're just not smart enough yet to sort it out.

POINTS 5 AND 7—ENTRY OF T_4 AND T_3 INTO CELLS AND CELL NUCLEI

On their own, thyroid hormones can cross most cell membranes, the walls separating tiny capillary blood vessels from the interiors of cells. Similar structures encase each cell's complement of chromosomes, forming its nucleus, which T_3 must enter to reach its receptor. Free diffusion, however, is a slow process and it doesn't even work in the brain because of the so-called blood-brain barrier. Thus, thyroid hormone entry into cells involves carrier mediation. A substance, probably a protein, "carries" T_4 through some microscopic doorway into its target cell, like a bride being lifted over the threshold. Furthermore, serum transport proteins may bind to cell surface receptors, in effect, handing off thyroid hormone to the described carrier-mediated process. There are also direct cell membrane receptors for T_4 and T_3.

A paper presented at the 2003 American Thyroid Association meeting in Palm Beach proposed that a genetic defect in T_3 transport was responsible for abnormal thyroid levels and mental retardation in two children. Beyond that tantalizing report, I am aware of no clinical disorders involving these points. Like point 4, this is a dim corner of the thyroid system. To presume we know enough about it, and to seriously claim nothing ever goes wrong there, is breathtakingly absurd.

POINT 6—CONVERSION OF T_4 TO T_3

In contrast, a process known to be riddled with problems is T_4 to T_3 peripheral conversion by the enzyme deiodinase—that is, the activation of the prohormone T_4 into the workhorse T_3. One reformist author, Dr. E. Denis Wilson, proposes that many patients with low-thyroid symptoms and normal blood tests have a defect at this level. *Wilson's thyroid syndrome* is the name given to this postulated disorder. As far as I know, no mainstream endocrinology text lists this condition, and the rare times I've heard it mentioned in lectures were solely for the purpose of ridicule. It is beyond the scope of this book to detail the controversies swirling about Wilson's thyroid syndrome—there are legitimate concerns—but I think mainstream medicine has been awfully quick to condemn the general notion of a thyroid disorder based on inadequate deiodinase action. In fact, I find it impossible to imagine such disorders don't exist.

Many things inhibit deiodinase and disrupt peripheral conversion. Any severe illness will block deiodinase action as part of what is probably an adaptive process wherein the ill body lowers its metabolic rate and conserves resources. That process, the euthyroid sick syndrome, has been the subject of countless articles, lectures, and textbook chapters for as long as I've been in medicine. Starvation is another potent inhibitor of deiodinase and the resulting fall in T_3 levels probably helps maintain nutritional resources. (Off-and-on dieting and skipping meals to lose weight may have similar effects on the thyroid system.)

The trace mineral selenium helps modulate endocrine processes throughout the body, including those of the thyroid system. Among the better understood roles of selenium is its necessary place in the structure of deiodinase, which is one of the few known selenium-containing proteins. Without selenium, deiodinase levels fall, possibly impairing T_4 to T_3 conversion. Other selenoproteins guard thyroid follicular cells from oxidative damage inflicted by chemical reactions involved in thyroid hormone synthesis. Their lack would eventually cause deficient T_4 and T_3 production (see point 3).

Numerous drugs block deiodinase function: glucocorticoids, iodine, or any medication containing iodine (the heart drug amiodarone is notorious), certain x-ray dyes, the antithyroid drug propylthiouracil, and the beta-blocker propranolol. Even beneficial antioxidants called flavonoids (found in tea, berries, apples, tomatoes, broccoli, carrots, and onions) have been implicated.

Of course, if glucocorticoid drugs block T_4 to T_3 conversion, then internal steroid excess due to Cushing's syndrome would do so as well. And what about our "soccer mom syndrome"—excessive cortisol production triggered by depression, anxiety, or chronic daily stress? And remember, steroid levels elevated by all these same factors also might cause occult central hypothyroidism (OCH). So, emotional stress, improperly managed, could create a low-grade state of steroid excess that might interfere with both T_4 production (due to OCH) and its activation to T_3 (via deiodinase inhibition). The result is a low-thyroid state in which TSH would not be elevated, T_4 and T_3 levels might not be obviously low, and the compensatory increase in T_3 usually seen in hypothyroidism doesn't happen—a cloaked disease.

I think of defective peripheral conversion as a form of thyroid hormone resistance (see points 8 and 9). It makes no difference how much of the prohormone T_4 is around. If enough of the real hormone, T_3, doesn't get made, the patient will look and feel hypothyroid.

I treated a woman a few years ago who came to me on thyroid hormone pills for hypothyroidism. She required higher doses than her primary-care doctor was willing to prescribe to get her TSH down to normal. I ended up pushing her dose upward to the point where her FT_4 was frankly high before she felt well and had a normal TSH. It turned out she was also taking large doses of propranolol, given by a neurologist for tremors. Propranolol is a drug that interferes with deiodinase. I speculated it was blocking her T_4 to T_3 conversion, causing her to be resistant to her thyroid pills. When her neurologist stopped the propranolol, she no longer needed the high doses of thyroid hormone.

POINTS 8 AND 9—THYROID HORMONE RECEPTORS

I lump together here the complex events that begin with the lock-and-key fitting of T_3 into its receptor and end with the multitude of possible thyroid hormone actions. The precise result of receptor activation depends on which target tissue we're talking about. In the brain, signal transmission in nerve cells might be enhanced. In the liver, toxins get broken down faster. In a skin sebaceous gland, more oil is secreted. In muscle, more oxygen is consumed and more work accomplished.

A hormone's receptor is its site of attachment onto, or within, a target cell, through which it orders some preprogrammed task to be performed. The T_3 receptor is located in the target cell's nucleus, attached to DNA, the genetic material itself. Do receptors always work perfectly? If not, they could be a potential cause of inadequate thyroid function that would defy the usual diagnostic rules. By now, you know it would cause me no heartburn to speculate about hormone receptors breaking down, but I don't need to speculate. This story goes back more than sixty years.

Hormone Resistance

In 1942, Fuller Albright (one of the fathers of modern endocrinology), working at Massachusetts General Hospital, described a condition called (believe it or not) pseudohypoparathyroidism. People with pseudohypoparathyroidism have low blood calcium levels and look to all the world like their parathyroid hormone (PTH) levels should also be low. But they're not—they're high.

High PTH should drive calcium levels up. Or, in the case of Dr. Albright's low-calcium patients, high PTH should restore calcium levels to normal. Pseudohypoparathyroidism was the first disease discovered to be caused by a hormone failing to act. Lots of hormone (PTH) gets made, but the expected response from the target cell doesn't happen. This phenomenon became known as hormone resistance. (The parathyroid glands and PTH, by the way, are part of a different hormone complex having nothing to do with our main subject, the thyroid system.)

There are many mechanisms of hormone resistance. The hormone might be altered so that it can't bind its receptor, or the receptor might be altered by genetic mutation with the same result. Something might be broken downstream in the signaling process that leads from receptor to hormone action. One result of a lack of target response is increased production of the hormone in question. The mother gland usually works normally in hormone resistance, the abnormality instead being in the target tissue. So, once the lack of effect is sensed, more hormone is pumped out in an appropriate attempt to overcome the resistance. Sometimes this succeeds, sometimes not, depending on the seriousness of the defect.

Thyroid Hormone Resistance

Does hormone resistance happen in the thyroid system? We've already mentioned bio-inactive TSH—this would be an example of thyrotropin (TSH) resistance. What about thyroid hormone itself? Such a disorder was discovered in 1967 by Dr. Samuel Refetoff, currently at the University of Chicago. More than 600 cases of Refetoff's syndrome (resistance to thyroid hormone or RTH) have been confirmed. Approximately 100 different genetic mutations altering the thyroid hormone receptor have been identified, all leading to a reduced response to T_3.

RTH is not supposed to cause low-thyroid symptoms. The defect is always partial, never complete, say the experts. When the pituitary gland senses the lack of thyroid effect, it spews out more TSH, resulting in more T_4 and T_3 production, eventually enough to overcome the resistance—in theory. I'm always suspicious of words like *always* and *never* in medicine.

People with RTH have high T_4 levels with normal or high TSH levels. The high T_4 has caused some with RTH to be incorrectly diagnosed with hyperthyroidism, and even wrongly treated for it. TSH levels that aren't low and the absence of high-thyroid symptoms should prevent such errors. This is another situation where good clinical evaluation should trump the numbers.

Now, this all sounds reasonably straightforward. Things get very confusing, though, when one tissue responds better to thyroid hormone than another. The mutation causing a specific person's RTH is present in every cell in the body, but some parts of the body are often more resistant than others. Assuming the amount of TSH released is based on some average level of responsiveness (it isn't—it's based on brain and pituitary responsiveness—but just suppose), then the amount of thyroid hormone produced would be too much for some organs, not enough for others, and just right for others still. Your body wouold react like Goldilocks in the three bears story.

Thus, patients with RTH can have a mix of signs and symptoms—some suggesting high thyroid, others suggesting low thyroid. If a person's genes carry an RTH mutation leaving her skin more resistant than her muscles, she might have hair loss and dry skin, but not muscle cramping. In fact, sometimes patients report what I describe back to them as a "mixed bag of symptoms": some sounding high and some low. The conclusion I typically draw is that their complaints probably aren't thyroid related. Otherwise, why would they be so contradictory? Patients usually agree with that logic, but what if some of these "mixed bag" people have RTH with a variable tissue response?

It is estimated that genetic RTH occurs once in every 50,000 births. Most think it uncommon to the point of absurdity, and many primary-care providers probably don't know it exists. RTH isn't even something many endocrinologists give a lot of thought to. Thus, it is a condition that is hardly ever going to come to mind as a serious diagnostic possibility.

But what if subtle RTH is more common than we think? If something is hard to diagnose and low on many doctors' lists of diseases to look for—and RTH meets those criteria—then the milder cases are bound to slip through the cracks. We know hypothyroidism is common and everybody knows to look for it, yet many cases get missed. That's the thyroid paradox. What on earth would make us think we pick up all or even a significant minority of RTH that's out there?

And let's not even get into primary hypothyroidism and RTH affecting the same individual—such as the case from Australia which was reported in the May 2006 issue of *Endocrine Practice*. How difficult might it be to diagnose and treat primary hypothyroidism adequately when RTH—with perhaps varying tissue hormone sensitivities—is monkeying around with the numbers?

Central versus Peripheral RTH

In RTH, tissues can vary in their responsiveness to thyroid hormone. What if the pituitary or hypothalamus differs dramatically in this respect from the rest of the body? You see, thyroid receptors in the pituitary and hypothalamus are the thyroid hormone sensors for the entire body. How much hormone gets made by the thyroid, under hypothalamic-pituitary-thyroid (HPT) axis control, is determined by how much hormone gets detected by the hypothalamus and pituitary glands. Put another way, how much hormone the body gets to work with is determined by central thyroid receptors. If the pituitary and/or hypothalamus disagree with the periphery (the rest of the body) on how much hormone is needed, it's "Houston, we have a problem" time.

According to Dr. Refetoff, peripheral tissues (skin, muscle, heart, liver, and so on) are *often* more thyroid-resistant than the pituitary. The reverse situation—the pituitary being more resistant than peripheral tissues (so-called central RTH)—is a rare cause of hyperthyroidism. The pituitary is blind to the adequate, if not excessive, thyroid levels in the bloodstream. The pituitary responds to what it perceives as a low-thyroid state by making more TSH, which worsens the hyperthyroidism.

But this book is about low thyroid, so it's the first situation that interests us. When the rest of the body has more resistance to thyroid hormone than the pituitary—what we'll call peripheral RTH—the pituitary is blind to the *deficiency* being experienced by most of the body. So, TSH doesn't change, and there is no increase in T_4 and T_3 production. That is, no effort is made to overcome the resistance. The person goes to her doctor with complaints sounding like hypothyroidism. Her TSH is checked and it's normal. Her FT_4 test, if done, may be normal or high, but it's not low. Whatever else this might be, it's not primary hypothyroidism, and that's where most doctors stop looking, or at least stop thinking it's the thyroid.

How do you avoid this trap? I might've stepped into this one dozens of times myself without realizing it—low-thyroid symptoms with a normal TSH. The best shot at making the diagnosis is if the FT_4 is high. A high FT_4 and a normal TSH should hardly ever coexist, so the tests should be repeated. Assuming similar results come back the second time, it's time to get an endocrinologist involved. The endocrinologist should make sure the TSH isn't falsely normal because of interfering antibodies. If that is not the case, then there has to be a defect in the HPT axis.

There are two HPT axis problems that could manifest with an FT_4 level that is truly high and a TSH that is truly *not* low. The first is hyperthyroidism due to TSH excess caused by either a tumor or central RTH, but these conditions generate high-thyroid symptoms. The second possibility, the one to consider if the patient is clinically hypothyroid, is peripheral RTH. The TSH is normal because the HPT axis is blind to the deficiency being experienced elsewhere, which causes the low-thyroid symptoms. The FT_4 is high, but not high enough to overcome the resistance.

Peripheral RTH could also yield a patient with low-thyroid complaints and an FT_4 and TSH that are both high. This person's pituitary or hypothalamus would be just a little more resistant to thyroid hormone than in the first example where the TSH was normal, but still less resistant than the periphery. Don't pull out too much hair trying to follow this. The important message is: thyroid disease can be a lot less simple than most doctors and practice guidelines give it credit for.

If both FT_4 and TSH are normal, how do we recognize peripheral RTH then? The only way is to realize the patient is clinically hypothyroid despite normal lab tests. In other words, symptoms should never be ignored even when tests are normal. They may or may not require treatment, but they should never be ignored.

The following are additional clues to occult peripheral RTH:

* A known family history of RTH (not very likely)

* Goiter (66% to 99% of RTH)

* Attention deficit hyperactivity disorder (ADHD; 40% to 60% of RTH)

* Learning disabilities (30%)

One of my patients is an ADHD teenager suffering what I suspect to be peripheral RTH. In order to make him normal—that is, not clinically hypothyroid—he requires doses of thyroid pills high enough to suppress his TSH below normal and raise his FT_4 above normal. It is my belief, as I explain during every visit to him and his mother, that he has RTH in which the pituitary is more responsive to thyroid hormone than are the peripheral tissues. Might his low TSH and high FT_4 be due simply to an overdose of thyroid hormone pills? That is a serious possibility, which is why I carefully question and examine him on each visit to be sure he is not being harmed by too much medicine.

So far, I've discussed RTH as if it were always genetic; in the usual sense of the term, it is. Earlier, though, I likened a drug blockade of T_4 to T_3 conversion to RTH, which would be an example of *acquired* RTH. Another example of acquired RTH was hinted at in a report that bisphenol A—a component of plastics widely used in everyday life—disrupts T_3 action at the level of target cells' DNA. And at the 2004 Endocrine Society meeting in New Orleans, research was presented suggesting that thyroid hormone pills chemically alter the thyroid hormone receptor, which might affect function and cause RTH.

A word of caution: in its various forms, RTH could be used to explain away almost any thyroid test result. Just plead RTH and the interpreting physician can morph data into whatever interpretation he or she wants. That makes thyroid resistance a risky diagnosis.

- *High FT_4 plus low TSH* might mean a person's Synthroid dose is too high and should be lowered, or it could be peripheral RTH. And if it is peripheral RTH, is the hormone dose low, high, or just right? It depends.

- *The lab work is perfect* might mean she's dosed just right, or maybe she has RTH that isn't compensating because the pituitary is less resistant than the rest of her body (again, peripheral RTH).

- *Both FT_4 and TSH are high* might mean she's not taking her hormone pills right—missing a bunch of doses, then loading up right before a doctor's appointment—or it might mean she has a TSH-secreting tumor, or central RTH.

My point is that a rampant reformist, or any doctor cowed by an insistent patient, could abuse the diagnosis of RTH and use it to justify inappropriate treatment. On the other hand, failing to recognize the possibility of RTH could leave a patient with real but atypical hypothyroidism twisting in the wind. It's comforting to believe that RTH is rare, because that gives doctors permission to ignore it. As soon as one allows for the possibility that more of it might be out there than was previously thought, then the well-ordered, compulsively neat world of conventional thyroidology flies apart. Under this scenario, no blood test is trustworthy without being correlated with signs and symptoms, which is as it should be.

POINT 10—THE BALANCING ACT

It is critically important to thyroid system operation that its central parts work in harmony with its peripheral ones. Yet, it is under-recognized—hardly ever recognized, really—that the system can be knocked off balance.

Consider the thyroid system like a playground teeter-totter. The hypothalamus and pituitary sit at one end, while serum transport proteins, deiodinases, and thyroid hormone receptors crowd onto the other. The fulcrum in the middle is the thyroid gland, which ties both ends together via its key role as the producer of thyroid hormone. Think of the teeter-totter analogy when imagining the normal negative feedback between the central end and the peripheral end of the system. When the peripheral end is low—when the thyroid hormone receptor is inadequately stimulated—the central end is high, producing more TSH to get more thyroid hormone secreted. As the peripheral end rises, the central end falls, and less TSH gets produced. And the cycle keeps repeating in perfect balance, like the teeter-totter going up and down, up and down.

What if the board bends or breaks? This would make both ends high at the same time or low at the same time, or introduce sluggishness in the response of one end to what the other end is doing. The system goes out of balance. Two things can do this:

- Failure of the pituitary or hypothalamus to sense what is happening at the other end (thyroid hormone resistance)

- Failure of the pituitary or hypothalamus to respond to what it does sense from the other end (central hypothyroidism)

The system can be broken and still be in balance. If the thyroid gland fails to make enough thyroid hormone—as in primary hypothyroidism—but the pituitary pumps out more TSH in response, then the central and peripheral ends are in balance. The patient may be sick and need treatment, but the system is balanced.

Anyone arguing that a TSH test alone is ever completely adequate for the diagnosis of hypothyroidism is saying that the system never goes out of balance. A normal TSH always means normal thyroid function, a high TSH always means low-thyroid function, and so forth. Clearly that is not the case. Central hypothyroidism and thyroid hormone resistance—both of which fill chapters in mainstream textbooks—are the nails in that coffin.

CHAPTER 7

THYROID REPLACEMENT 101

Thyroid hormone's use as a drug dates to 1891, when sheep thyroid extract was injected into a woman suffering with severe myxedema (a largely obsolete term for hypothyroidism). This was the first instance of hormone replacement therapy, predating the use of insulin for diabetes by three decades. A year later, oral consumption of sautéed sheep thyroid was found to be an effective alternative to shots. Tablets formed from the dried (desiccated) thyroids of domesticated animals (mainly swine) soon followed and remain in limited use today. The Mayo Clinic's Edward Kendall chemically isolated thyroxine (T_4) on Christmas Day in 1914. His compound was patented and unsuccessfully marketed, because it was more expensive and less effective than existing animal-derived products. This early failure of pure T_4 pills partly explains the persisting belief in some circles that desiccated animal thyroid (known as thyroid USP and marketed under the trade name Armour Thyroid) is the superior way to treat hypothyroidism. The problem with Dr. Kendall's preparation, though, was that it was poorly absorbed from the intestinal tract, an issue resolved long ago by using the sodium salt, rather than the free-acid form of the molecule.

Mass production of synthetic T_4 in the form of levothyroxine (LT_4) came by the late 1940s. This development made pure T_4 treatment economically competitive with thyroid USP. The first commercially available LT_4, Synthroid, came to market in 1958, but it wasn't until the mid-1970s that LT_4 started replacing thyroid USP on a large scale. Why did this occur? It was established in the 1950s that there were two major thyroid hormones, T_4 and T_3. A synthetic T_3-only pill (liothyronine, or LT_3) actually beat Synthroid to market in 1956. But neither LT_4 nor LT_3 were often used alone because it was assumed hypothyroid patients needed both to normalize their thyroid status. And since thyroid USP contained both (because the animal organs it was made from did), it remained the preferred thyroid pill.

Everything changed after four landmark papers were published between 1970 and 1973. These articles revealed (1) the existence of peripheral conversion of T_4 to T_3, (2) that 80 percent of blood T_3 came from that peripheral conversion, (3) that T_4 by itself was less potent than T_3, and (4) that LT_4 used alone maintained stable serum levels of both T_4 and T_3. As a result, by the time I entered medical school in 1983, few still took thyroid USP and Synthroid was the industry giant.

End of story? I'm afraid not. As people were being switched *en masse* from thyroid USP to LT_4, it became immediately apparent that some of them didn't feel as well. And so was born the myth of thyroid USP as a martyred *natural* drug that "evil" doctors are determined to keep people from getting, or so some reformists would have us believe. More on that controversy later.

Thyroid hormone treatment comes in two varieties: suppression and replacement. Thyroid suppression therapy is the use of thyroid pills to lower TSH levels for the purpose of shrinking or stabilizing goiters, nodules, or thyroid cancer. Since hypothyroidism, not goiters, nodules, and so on, is the concern of this book, I will not further discuss suppression therapy. Much of what will be said, however, applies to both suppression and replacement. Thyroid replacement therapy (TRT) is given to correct thyroid hormone deficiency—hypothyroidism. Its usual goal is the achievement of a normal TSH (again, that problematic word *normal*).

As of this writing, four brand-name LT_4 products are available in the United States—Synthroid, Levoxyl, Levothroid, and Unithroid—as well as several generic products. A few years ago, the U.S. Food and Drug Administration (FDA) set off a controversy when it threatened withdrawal from the United States market of several LT_4 products never officially approved—only because, as a group, thyroid pills predated the Federal Food, Drug, and Cosmetic Act of 1938. That law for the first time required pharmaceutical companies to prove their drugs were safe before selling them to the public. Drugs in existence prior to the legislation were "grandfathered in," which is how Synthroid and the others avoided the regulations for so long. The recent hullabaloo occurred after quality-assurance concerns led the FDA to order that all versions of LT_4 be submitted for review. The maker of Synthroid kicked and screamed a lot about this at the time, generating some negative press now being wrongly held against the product by some reformists. At this point, however, the issues are moot. All previously available name brands, including Synthroid, have earned FDA approval.

BRANDED VERSUS GENERIC DRUGS

Another persisting controversy centers around the "Synthroid lawsuit." A class-action suit was filed in 1996 against the manufacturer of Synthroid. It alleged that Knoll Pharmaceuticals (Abbott Laboratories, Synthroid's current producer, was never involved) unfairly tried to conceal evidence that generic forms of LT_4 were just as good as the more expensive brand-name pills. A settlement was reached. The important point for the millions taking Synthroid, then and now, is that the suit was over business practices and never involved a concern for the quality and safety of the product.

By the way, the study alleging that all forms of LT_4 were equivalent—the one at the core of the Synthroid lawsuit—reached its conclusions based on total T_4 (TT_4) testing only. I've already given you my opinion that TT_4 tests used alone are virtually worthless. Information given to me by the manufacturer of Synthroid (take that with as big a grain of salt as you want, but I don't disbelieve the data—especially since it has subsequently been published in a peer-reviewed journal) purports to detail the TSH levels from that study, which should be more indicative of how patients actually faired when switching brands. And those TSH levels were all over the map.

The debate goes on. The FDA recently declared some generic products to be equivalent to branded preparations like Synthroid. This has resulted in an epidemic of patients being switched by their pharmacists (often without their doctors' knowledge) from a brand-name product they've been stable on and happy with, possibly for years, to a cheaper generic drug. In Tennessee, a recent state law meant to cut healthcare costs made it easier for pharmacies to do this. In my clinic, in some cases, such changes from brand name to generic have made no difference. In others, I firmly believe the ill-advised switch to a generic product, without my consent (what I consider to be an unconscionable violation of my prescriptive authority), has resulted in patients' meticulously balanced thyroid levels being thrown out of control, requiring more adjustments, more blood testing, and more office visits.

The problem is that LT_4 products made by different manufacturers have different bioavailabilities. Bioavailability refers to how much of the swallowed dose of a drug actually ends up in the bloodstream in a usable form. For thyroid hormone, in the eyes of the practicing physician, the best determinants of bioavailability are resulting TSH levels and symptom relief. Dose X of Synthroid might result in a different TSH level than dose X of Unithroid. My own thyroid levels became noticeably higher on Levoxyl than on the same dose of Synthroid (my TSH *and* my symptoms changed), but that doesn't mean there's anything wrong with Levoxyl. It means that if you switch brands, retesting and possibly dose adjustments are required. This is consistent with published guidelines from the American Thyroid Association and FDA-approved labeling of these drugs. So, unless you like doctors' offices and needle sticks, I suggest staying with one brand. *Which* one doesn't matter.

Unfortunately, the FDA uses neither TSH levels nor symptoms to compare the bioavailabilities of thyroid pills. Like the flawed study I cited, it looks at TT_4 levels. Mainstream endocrinology has serious disagreements with the FDA about their scientific methods, conclusions, and actions on this issue. Unfortunately, the government agency has virtually ignored the prevailing opinion of thyroid medical experts. You should be concerned and wary that your pharmacy might try to give you a generic drug that your doctor might not want you to have. I agree with the joint statement from the Endocrine Society, the American Association of Clinical Endocrinologists, and the American Thyroid Association, issued in June 2004, in response to the FDA action. It urged doctors to avoid generic LT_4 products and reiterated the need for repeat thyroid function testing any time brands are switched. Additionally, the respected and unbiased *Medical Letter*, in its issue of September 27, 2004, advised not introducing the variable of generic substitution into the already complex world of thyroid prescribing.

To be clear, none of this says that any one company's product is flawed. The issue is switching back and forth. This is nothing new. I remember sitting in a medical school classroom in 1988—long before I was diagnosed with hypothyroidism, or had ever treated a patient, or even considered the thyroid a particular area of interest—and being taught by a pharmacology professor that generic substitutions for brand-name products were acceptable. With two exceptions, one of which was Synthroid.

It should be obvious why generic LT_4 is condemned. If you walk into a pharmacy with a generic prescription, you can be given any manufacturer's product. No problem, until you go back for a refill. Then you might get a different company's LT_4. On the next refill, you get a third brand. The only way I can be sure my patient gets the same brand every time is to specify a brand and mark "Do Not Substitute" or "Dispense as Written" on the prescription pad. I only prescribe generic thyroid pills after a face-to-face discussion of these issues with my patient, and he or she has convinced me that the cost savings (the only legitimate reason to do it) would be significant to him or her.

SYNTHETIC VERSUS NATURAL

Thyroid USP (brand name, Armour Thyroid) is favored by some reformists as a "natural" alternative to manufactured drugs like Synthroid. This argument is weak since the T_4 contained in thyroid USP is exactly the same molecule as the T_4 in Synthroid. The former was made inside an animal, while the latter was made in a factory. I'm unsure why that matters provided the molecules are the same, but I personally prefer taking a drug coming out of a sterile factory rather than an exploited animal.

Where thyroid USP does indisputably differ from Synthroid, Levoxyl, and the others is that it contains both T_4 and T_3, which may give thyroid USP an advantage in those possibly needing T_3 in addition to T_4. Thyroid USP is also enriched (or contaminated) with the minor metabolites of thyroid hormone (T_1, T_2, reverse T_3, and various thyroid hormone conjugates). If these substances are important, then the natural product would have an advantage, because this mix would be hard for industry to duplicate. An open mind should be maintained, but to date research has not shown the minor metabolites to have any significant therapeutic impact. They are thought to be metabolic garbage.

But—it is fervently argued by some—thyroid USP is natural. I assume *natural* is supposed to be a buzzword for *safer*. If so, I can't see how a drug containing more active ingredients can possibly be safer than a drug containing a single well-understood one. The natural product may or may not be more effective, but there's no way it's safer. And thyroid USP is not entirely natural: it comes from an animal, but Forest Pharmaceuticals processes Armour Thyroid in their factory, not in a native hut. According to the *Physicians' Desk Reference*, its ingredients include calcium stearate, dextrose microcrystalline cellulose, sodium starch glycolate, and opadry white. Don't ask me what any of that stuff is, but I doubt it came from the pig.

Are natural substances necessarily safer, incidently? No. Curare, a deadly South American arrow poison, is brewed from the stems, roots, bark, and leaves of several Amazonian plant species. But it is far from safe. Natural or synthetic, if a drug is strong enough to help, it's strong enough to hurt. In my opinion, there is way too much panic these days over the dangers of prescription drugs. They are all dangerous! It's the physician's job to weigh the risks versus the benefits, explain them to the patient, and, if a drug is started, monitor for good and bad results. The bottom line: thyroid USP may or may not be superior to LT_4 in some people needing thyroid replacement, but "natural" has nothing to do with it.

T_4 VERSUS T_3

Pure T_4 therapy is the current standard among conventional physicians.

Some argue, however, that T_3 is preferable, either alone or in combination with T_4. Some argue that LT_4 is next to worthless (the same pundits who vilify blood testing). Their logic is simple: if T_3 is more potent than T_4, and if T_4 has little activity on its own, doesn't it make sense for hypothyroid patients to take T_3?

Perhaps. To mimic normal physiology, a pill containing a mixture of T_4 and T_3 comes the closest, since the thyroid gland manufactures both hormones. But most T_3 in the body comes from peripheral conversion. The long-standing mainstream rationale has been that we don't have to give T_3 because the body will make however much it needs out of the T_4 it's given. It's even debatable whether increasing serum T_3 with a hormone pill has much effect inside cells, where deiodinases play a role in establishing just the right T_3 levels.

By the way, it's not a given that a low-thyroid patient doesn't get T_3 from her own gland. Hypothyroidism means a patient can't manufacture enough hormone to meet her needs. She might be able, though, to meet 20 percent, 50 percent, even 80 percent of those requirements. And since the normal thyroid doesn't make much T_3 anyway, a lot of low-thyroid patients may still make plenty. That's probably why, in my professional and personal experience, most patients do fine with LT_4 therapy alone. The people more likely to benefit from T_3 therapy are those who have suffered a complete or near-complete destruction of the thyroid, from long-standing Hashimoto's thyroiditis or total surgical removal.

There is no "one size fits all" thyroid replacement strategy. Nevertheless, most doctors writing thyroid prescriptions never think beyond LT_4 alone, just as many never think beyond TSH in the diagnostic phase of hypothyroidism management. I believe, in a minority of cases, the severity or underlying cause of the hypothyroidism might make combination T_4/T_3 therapy preferable. Also, some of the more esoteric disorders, such as resistance to thyroid hormone or impaired T_4 to T_3 conversion, might do better with dual therapy.

The T_4/T_3 question is a swinging pendulum. For the first eighty years of the TRT era, combined therapy in the form of thyroid USP was the standard. Between the 1950s and the 1970s, the pendulum swung back—

slowly at first, then rapidly—almost all the way to LT_4 alone. Now, perhaps, we're seeing a slow swing the opposite way.

THE PROS AND CONS OF DIFFERING THYROID REPLACEMENT STRATEGIES

We will now detail the three alternative ways of delivering thyroid hormone pharmacologically: levothyroxine (LT_4), liothyronine (LT_3), or a combination.

LT_4 Only

Levothyroxine alone is the most frequent way mainstream doctors, myself included, do thyroid replacement therapy (TRT). This is what I personally take as well. Whether in the form of Synthroid, Levoxyl, Levothroid, Unithroid, or a generic, LT_4 is a single drug, and dealing with one hormone pill rather than two, assuming it does the job, appeals to my KISS (Keep It Simple, Stupid) philosophy. Simplicity is especially important when therapy is likely to be lifelong, as in the case with TRT. Also, since many dose sizes are produced, LT_4 can be adjusted easily and precisely. This is critical since changes as small as 25–50 micrograms (mcg) can significantly alter TSH levels and metabolic rate.

Because it is less potent, LT_4 is less likely than liothyronine (LT_3) to cause hyperthyroid side effects, yet it provides the raw material the body needs to "naturally" manufacture T_3. LT_4 is long-acting, meaning it only has to be taken once daily, and serum levels hold pretty steady. Consequently, drug levels don't drop much when a dose is missed or delayed. If a person without a thyroid gland stopped taking LT_4 today, it would take a week for her free thyroxine level to drop halfway. That means people should feel no different, say, two hours after taking Unithroid than they did before. Also, they shouldn't notice anything if they're a little late taking their pill. Occasionally, a patient tells me about feeling bad until scarfing down that thyroid pill each morning, and then feeling fine. Pharmacologically, it's not supposed to happen that way, but people are different and I don't want to be too dogmatic. Nevertheless, reports such as that suggest to me a psychological dependence on the pill rather than actual drug effect. (Don't confuse LT_4 and LT_3 on this point: LT_3 is fast-acting and people definitely notice when they do or don't take it.)

To summarize, the good things about LT_4-only TRT are as follows:

- One kind of pill to take

- Once-a-day dosing

- Large variety of doses available

- Stable blood levels and more leeway if a dose is missed

- Relatively safe

- Mimics natural function by providing T_4 to be made into T_3 by the body

What are the downsides? LT_4 does not provide T_3 to those who need it, which is a controversial point even among mainstreamists. Along the same lines, being less potent, LT_4 may not correct hypothyroid signs and symptoms as quickly and effectively as LT_3 in some patients. In fact, when LT_4-treated patients with a normal TSH were compared to people with no thyroid disease history, the treated low-thyroid people felt worse: 37 percent had multiple complaints versus 25 percent of controls. Commenting on this paper, Dr. Robert Utiger, of Harvard Medical School, speculated that either the LT_4 dose was inadequate or the patients needed to be given LT_3 as well. He concluded: "We need to focus less on serum TSH values and think more about how to treat patients with hypothyroidism in new ways." Still, the positives for LT_4-only TRT outnumber the negatives. It may not be for everybody, but it's a good entry-level thyroid therapy.

LT_3 Only

Doctors sometimes use LT_3 alone for short periods to prepare thyroid cancer patients for radioactive iodine treatments. Also, LT_3-only therapy has long been used by psychiatrists to augment antidepressants in severe depression. Synthetic T_3-only TRT, however, has never been popular with thyroidologists for routine use. The prevailing theory in the 1970s, when patients were being switched from thyroid USP in droves, was that T_3 supplements weren't needed: Mother Nature would always manufacture it in just the right amount out of T_4. To a large degree, this opinion persists. But beyond the question of whether T_3 supplements are needed, there are definite practical disadvantages to LT_3-only TRT.

For example, the greater potency of LT_3 equates to an increased risk of hyperthyroid side effects. Its shorter duration of action means that hormone levels fluctuate. Plus, two or three doses per day are needed to maintain round-the-clock benefits. Even then, hormone levels may unavoidably drift out of the desired range for a few hours at a time.

The primary LT_3 product in the United States is Cytomel. This pill comes in only three sizes—5, 25, and 50 mcg—versus, for instance, Levoxyl's twelve dosages. That means if doses are to be precisely adjusted, it is often impossible to get by with a single LT_3 pill, which is almost always possible with LT_4. So, besides having to take it two or three times daily, each dose may be composed of two tablets or a half tablet that the patient has to break. These minor issues become major ones when you consider that thyroid replacement therapy is usually required every day for the rest of one's life. And that's just the hassle factor. What about mistakes? The more complicated the plan, the more likely a patient is to take the wrong dose.

Despite these concerns, some reformists do promote the use of LT_3 alone, either in the form of Cytomel or as specially compounded sustained-release preparations. Often they recommend doses higher than most doctors are comfortable with. Some suggest ignoring suppressed TSH levels, which most of us equate with dangerous thyroid excess. I have presented scenarios where an undetectable TSH in a patient on TRT would not indicate excess—central hypothyroidism or some forms of thyroid hormone resistance, for example. But very low TSH levels get my respect: they are potentially dangerous for most people and should be avoided unless circumstances strongly suggest otherwise. A reformist might correctly argue low TSH levels aren't *always* bad, but neither can we assume they are *always* safe. Some reformist authors confidently report nirvana-like results using high-dose T_3-only TRT, with no ill effects. Perhaps that *is* their experience, and their perception, but in the spirit of "first do no harm" I want to know a lot more about their research before buying in. First, I don't know any drug on the planet—synthetic or natural—that is perfectly free of side effects. Remember, strong enough to help means strong enough to hurt. And call me a cynic, but I consider any claims of perfect results to be suspicious. More specifically, though, some reformists seem oblivious to even the potential danger of hyperthyroidism.

Yet, it was shown by the landmark Framingham study that elderly men with undetectable TSH levels carried a threefold higher risk for atrial fibrillation, a dangerous type of irregular heartbeat that can cause a stroke. Also, high thyroid increases the heart's workload and, like a biceps muscle, working heart muscle thickens, which eventually interferes with proper filling and emptying of its pumping chambers. Osteoporosis is the other worry: numerous studies show that, at least in older women, low TSH levels are associated with lower bone density, and low bone density is associated with hip fracture. Not all studies agree that hyperthyroidism begets fractures, but the weight of evidence suggests danger. If you're not an older woman, the bone risk of high-dose LT_3 may not be of much significance. The same is true of the heart problems if you're less than fifty years old. But I don't think these concerns should be completely ignored at any age.

In my opinion, it is never justified to treat a hypothyroid patient with any form of T_3 hormone alone for extended periods, especially in large doses. You need look no further than nature to see the flaw in T_3-only TRT. Our own thyroid glands mostly make T_4, with only a little T_3. In thyroid replacement, doesn't it make sense to provide what the thyroid gland was mostly providing? In other words, T_4.

You might argue that in a case of blocked peripheral conversion, where the person makes plenty of T_4 but can't activate it to T_3, giving T_3 is reasonable. I agree that situation comes up, but it's not something we know a lot about in the outpatient setting. The only defective peripheral conversion situation that has been studied to any degree is the euthyroid sick syndrome, which occurs only in critically ill patients—and it remains controversial, even then, whether LT$_3$ is useful and safe. Additionally, research has suggested that LT$_3$ supplementation can be helpful in certain heart surgeries. But neither the euthyroid-sick nor the heart-surgery situation apply outside the hospital. Treatment in an intensive-care patient is always short-lived, a matter of days or weeks. Any experience in the hospitalized patient is, therefore, irrelevant when we talk about longer-term, perhaps lifelong, treatment.

When it comes to treating outpatient peripheral conversion defects, like the postulated Wilson's syndrome, doctors need to have a reliable way of diagnosing the problem before proceeding, and to be reasonably sure that the cure isn't worse than the disease. For now, there is no peer-reviewed research showing T$_3$-only TRT to be safe, effective, and necessary. And while I have advocated in these pages the rather aggressive use of LT$_4$ treatment—sometimes in the face of peer-reviewed research—I think safety concerns obviate using LT$_3$ in the same manner. Might I be denying my patient potentially helpful therapy by taking this position? Yes, but my first obligation is to do no harm. *Primum non nocere*.

T$_4$/T$_3$ Cocktail

Even the stodgy mainstream is riding the pendulum partway back to the T$_3$ side. A resurgence of interest in combination T$_4$/T$_3$ therapy was sparked by a 1999 *New England Journal of Medicine* article entitled "Effects of Thyroxine as Compared with Thyroxine Plus Triiodothyronine in Patients with Hypothyroidism." Thirty-three low-thyroid patients were tested after taking LT$_4$ alone, and again after taking 50 mcg less than their original dose of LT$_4$ plus 12.5 mcg of LT$_3$ daily. The researchers found improvement in mood and neuropsychological testing after the two-drug course.

Not everyone is on board, however. At the Endocrine Society meeting in Philadelphia, the above-mentioned paper was discussed by one of the most knowledgeable experts on hypothyroidism. He criticized it on several technical points and challenged its conclusions. Two recent studies published in the *Journal of Clinical Endocrinology and Metabolism* supported his position, failing to prove any benefit from LT$_4$/LT$_3$ therapy over LT$_4$

alone. An editorial acknowledged that some patients find LT_4-only TRT unsatisfactory, but said more study was needed to find the solution.

Many doctors are keeping an open mind and use LT_4 plus LT_3 in some patients. Certainly combination therapy is more palatable to the mainstream than LT_3-only TRT, because it mimics what the thyroid actually does. The questions are: Who needs the added cost and complexity, and how much of each hormone should be given?

T_4-plus-T_3 TRT can be done two ways: a fixed-dose composite pill or two separate prescriptions, one for LT_4 and one for LT_3. I usually do the latter, prescribing both Synthroid or an equivalent, plus Cytomel in the exact doses I want. I generally prefer to avoid pharmaceutical products containing more than one drug in a single pill, because I like to be able to adjust the dosage of the different components separately. This is especially a concern with thyroid replacement therapy, where precise dosing is key.

There are fixed-dose combination TRT products available. Already mentioned is the animal-derived thyroid USP (Armour Thyroid). Another is liotrix (trade name Thyrolar), a synthetic T_4-plus-T_3 pill. In two decades of patient-care experience, I cannot recall ever seeing Thyrolar used by anyone. Both thyroid USP and liotrix come in a variety of dosage sizes, but fewer than the LT_4-only products. Also, the ratio of T_4 to T_3 is the same regardless of dose and—in the opinion of mainstreamists—all contain too much T_3.

According to the *Physicians' Desk Reference*, Armour Thyroid (thyroid USP) contains 38 mcg of T_4 and 9 mcg of T_3 per 60 milligram (mg) tablet. To give 76 mcg of T_4 per day (the low end of the average range of daily T_4 secretion from the normal human thyroid), the manufactured formulation would require someone to take 120 mg of Armour Thyroid, containing 18 mcg of T_3. But the normal thyroid only secretes 4–6 mcg of T_3 in a day, according to published data. So, to give a natural amount of T_4 with Armour Thyroid, I have to give a threefold overdose of T_3. It's roughly the same situation for Thyrolar. In my opinion, if the same thing can be accomplished with two separate drugs, which allows more freedom to prescribe as much or as little of each hormone as seems appropriate for the individual, that's the best way to go.

As composite pills go, thyroid USP is as good as any. It has a high degree of patient acceptance: many swear by it, refusing to switch to LT_4, or begging to go back after switching. One reason for this loyalty, I think, is a sort of "high" patients get from the burst of T_3 action in the few hours after dosing. People such as myself who have only taken LT_4 don't miss this because we've never experienced it. So, to some extent the love affair with thyroid USP may be an addiction to the "feel good" effects of mild hyperthyroidism. Theoretically, a physical dependence could develop as well. Patients used to getting T_3 by mouth may lose full deiodinase capability and be less able to naturally convert T_4 to T_3. In other words, a patient on thyroid USP may develop a peripheral conversion defect caused by the drug itself, which might make it difficult or impossible to switch to LT_4.

I should confess to having seldom prescribed thyroid USP, partly because of the concerns taught me by the mainstream, which, despite being older and wiser, I still largely share. I literally was never taught to use it, just to stamp it out. I can give thyroid USP when pressed to, just not with the honed skill and confidence I enjoy with LT_4. The same will be true of most doctors who started practice after the mid-1970s.

BASICS OF THYROID REPLACEMENT THERAPY

Eight to 12 million Americans take thyroid pills, creating a $600-million annual market. In 2001, Synthroid was the third best-selling prescription drug in the United States with 43.5 million prescriptions written. Like its diagnosis, treatment of low thyroid is fraught with difficulties and subtleties. The prescribing of levothyroxine (LT_4) is a daily occurrence in doctors' offices worldwide, specialist and nonspecialist alike. Some do it well, others less so.

- How high a dose should be given to start? The most common mistake I see is too little.

- How much should the dose be changed if levels aren't right? The most common mistake I see is too much. Every few months, I hear of a doctor doubling a dose—say, from 100 to 200 mcg—when the correct adjustment most often would be to increase it in 12.5 mcg or 25 mcg increments. The patient is then told it's a mystery why she can't be controlled better.

- How soon should blood levels be rechecked after starting or changing a dose? The most common mistake is to check them too soon—that is, before about five or six weeks. My mother used to say, "Patience is a virtue." That is definitely true with thyroid replacement therapy.

- If the goal of therapy is, by definition, a normal TSH level, what if my doctor says my dose is right because my tests are normal, but I still feel rotten? This sounding familiar?

A FIELD GUIDE TO THYROID PILLS

Unless otherwise stated, I will refer to LT_4-only treatment. LT_4 is actually an extremely potent medication, more than even most doctors give it credit for. *Potency* is a measure of how much effect, gram for gram, you get from a drug. If drug A treats the same disease as drug B, but drug A is one hundredfold more potent, that means 1 mcg of drug A will have the same effect as 100 mcg of drug B. Because LT_4 is so potent, it doesn't take much of a dose change to see a clinical and biochemical effect. That's why doubling LT_4 from 25 mcg to 50 mcg per day might be okay, but from 100 mcg to 200 mcg usually isn't.

If you're taking LT_4, examine your bottle. There's lot's of good information to be found there. First, check which brand you have. Make sure it's what your doctor ordered. It should be the same brand you got last time and the time before that, unless a change was discussed or you know you're getting a generic. It's not that your brand can never be changed, but you need to be sure it's not changed unintentionally. I've had patients get upset thinking they'd been given a generic when "levothyroxine" appears on the label. That *is* the generic name for the drug, but it may still be a brand-name product. Make sure the proper trade name (Synthroid, Levoxyl, Levothroid, or Unithroid) also appears somewhere on the label. But, if it says something like "levothyroxine, generic for Synthroid," you are getting a generic. (It is my understanding that the name of the actual product contained in the bottle is supposed to appear most boldly on the label.) If you are unsure, ask your doctor or pharmacist.

You should also be able to identify the brand by looking at the tablets. Synthroids are round and have the word *Synthroid* printed on one side. Levoxyls are the easiest to identify: they have an oblong butterfly shape and also carry the drug's name. Levothroid pills are oval, while Unithroid is round like Synthroid but has different printing.

The strength, which you should also check, will be on the label in either milligrams (mg) or micrograms (mcg). A milligram is 1,000 times more than a microgram. Thus, 0.1 mg is the same as 100 mcg. All LT_4 brand-name products are available in the same strengths, color-coded for easy identification: 25 mcg (orange), 50 mcg (white), 75 mcg (violet), 88 mcg (olive), 100 mcg (yellow), 112 mcg (rose), 125 mcg (brown), 137 mcg (dark blue), 150 mcg (blue), 175 mcg (lilac), 200 mcg (pink), and 300 mcg (green).

HOW TO TAKE IT

Taking LT_4 is pretty easy: put it in your mouth, sip some water, and swallow. Seriously, swallowing the pill regularly and reliably every day is more than half the battle. Sometimes, a patient facing TRT tells me how they've heard thyroid replacement is hard to get adjusted correctly. In my experience, after treating thousands of people over the past seventeen years (myself included), that simply isn't true. Thyroid replacement is remarkably easy for most people. Exceptions to that rule boil down to two problems: doctors dosing incorrectly (like leaping from 100 to 200 mcg) or people not taking the hormone pills as instructed.

Not everyone is disciplined about taking medications correctly. They're forgetful or busy or don't think it matters that much. Fortunately, LT_4 has a half-life of almost a week. This means it hangs around in the body long enough that you can make up for accidentally missed doses. Take it later in the day, or two pills the next day, or three pills the day after that if two days have been skipped.

When should LT_4 be taken? This is rarely a critical issue. It is more important to take your pills every day than it is to take them at a certain time. On the other hand, you need to establish some kind of habit if you're going to remember to do this daily for the rest of your life. Some people prefer taking hormone pills first thing in the morning, some at bedtime, and some with meals. For the most part, anything is fine. If you press me, though, I'll tell you the best time to take LT_4 is first thing in the morning on an empty stomach. Food can block absorption of thyroid hormone, as can certain drugs, so taking it on an empty stomach will result in higher serum levels of T_4 than dosing on a full stomach. I don't often make a big deal about this because I can compensate for any interference by prescribing a higher dose, as long as the patient is consistent—that is, takes her pill about the same time every day. On the other hand, if I'm having unusual difficulty getting a patient's levels up, or if they fluctuate a lot, then I will suggest she take her pills immediately upon arising. Strictly speaking, she should then wait a half hour before eating. In real life, though, I recommend—and this is what I do myself—that she just take the pill, then go through her regular morning routine of, say, showering and dressing, and then get breakfast without worrying about the timing. It'll be close enough.

Contrary to the above suggestions, research was presented at the 2004 Endocrine Society meeting in New Orleans claiming that absorption of LT_4 was better and TSH levels were lower in people taking their pills at bedtime. Bottom line: you can feel free to take thyroid hormone whenever it is most convenient. If a problem arises, then you can try a different approach.

Because of the variety of strengths available, most patients can swallow exactly the thyroid dose needed in the form of a single pill. When it does become necessary to give a dose that isn't manufactured—say, 62.5 mcg—there are a number of tricks. The patient can take a white 50 mcg one day and a purple 75 mcg the next and keep alternating. Or take two and a half 25 mcg pills every day, or a 50 mcg and half a 25 mcg, or half of a 125 mcg. She can even take one 50 mcg pill per day, Monday through Friday, and two 50 mcg pills on Saturday and Sunday, which will average out to 64 mcg per day over the week: (50 mcg × 9 tablets per week) ÷ 7 days = 64 mcg per day. Yet another option: take 75 mcg every day except Sunday—six instead of seven tablets per week. I try to avoid these games when possible, because they can cause confusion. We always want to keep dosing instructions as simple as we can.

Most people have heard of half-life in the context of radioactivity. It's the rate at which a radioactive substance sheds energy until it's no longer radioactive—specifically, the amount of time it takes for half of a mass of radioactive material to decay. Pharmacological half-life is how long it takes the concentration of a chemical in the bloodstream to drop by half; this occurs largely via breakdown in the liver and/or excretion through the kidneys. LT_4 has a long half-life—almost a week. A drug needs to be administered at least once per half-life in order to achieve and maintain stable serum levels. Theoretically, then, a person could take seven LT_4 pills weekly instead of one pill daily. For most folks, though, it's easier to get into the habit of once daily, so that's what is generally recommended. But since the total micrograms taken over a week is more important than the total taken in a day, a person can get away with skipping pills or taking an extra on Sunday, or taking different doses on alternating days (as I outlined above).

Here's an example. Karen's thyrotropin (TSH) level is a little high (that is, thyroid levels are low) on Synthroid at 150 mcg per day. Next time around, it's a little low (thyroid levels are high) on a dose of 175 mcg per day. I'd probably next try 162.5 mcg per day. Karen could alternate 150 mcg and 175 mcg pills, but she may not want to make two copayments to the pharmacy for two prescriptions. What I do is figure the total weekly dose equivalent to 162.5 mcg per day: That's $162.5 \times 7 = 1,137.5$ mcg. Then, I figure how many doses of an existing tablet, such as 175 mcg, it would take to equal the needed weekly dose: $1,137.5 \div 175 = 6.5$. Six and a half doses of 175 mcg per week will give Karen the right amount of thyroid hormone. So, Karen can take one 175 mcg tablet every day Monday through Saturday, and a half pill on Sunday.

It's hard to remember to take pills and harder to remember to do something different once a week, but one of the keys to successful TRT is consistency. Nobody's perfect with thyroid pills—even me—but it is critical to take the right dose on the right day most of the time.

MONKEY WRENCHES

A number of drugs reduce gastrointestinal absorption of LT_4 and should not be taken within two hours of it. These include iron and iron-containing vitamins, calcium, and aluminum-hydroxide antacids like Mylanta. Soy products also interfere. It was recently reported that stomach acid is required for optimal LT_4 absorption. Therefore, proton-pump inhibitors (potent anti-ulcer and acid reflux drugs) like Prilosec, Prevacid, and Nexium, which decrease acid production, unintentionally decrease the bioavailability of LT_4. Taking Synthroid and, say, Nexium two or more hours apart won't help this problem, because the acid-lowering effect of the latter is persistent. The dose of LT_4 needed to achieve the desired TSH level in these ulcer and reflux patients will simply be higher and no special action need be taken by you as the patient.

Higher doses of LT_4 are also generally required after weight gain and during pregnancy. In pregnancy, thyroid needs may increase as much as 50 percent. This is especially problematic since mildly low thyroid levels in pregnancy have been linked to a reduced IQ in the child. Very cold climates also seem to increase LT_4 consumption because of an increased need for body heat (U.S. Army researchers have dubbed this the "polar T_3 syndrome").

My own research and experience suggest that regular exercise and better fitness increase thyroid hormone need. That is, a 150-pound triathlete probably needs more LT_4 to maintain the same TSH level than a 150-pound couch potato. About nine years ago, I was running and weight lifting several times a week. I was taking 163 mcg of Synthroid per day at that time. After I left the Air Force, I stopped weight lifting for a while and decreased my running by about half. When I became less active and less physically fit, the dose I needed dropped to only 137 mcg per day. I later started to walk, run, and lift more frequently again and my dose went up to 150 mcg. Across all these years and different doses, my TSH level has been consistent, I've felt fine, and my weight has stayed almost the same. The only difference has been the amount and intensity of exercise.

THYROID REPLACEMENT AND THE HEART

Thyroid hormone increases the heart's workload and appetite for oxygen. In people with coronary heart disease (CHD; blockages in the arteries supplying blood to the heart), this can trigger chest pain or even a heart attack. In other words, TRT in some people might promote heart problems. We especially worry about this in the elderly.

But the thyroid-heart connection goes beyond mere treatment side effects. Low thyroid, the medical condition itself, can both cause and mask heart problems. Hypothyroidism increases artery-clogging cholesterol levels, *causing* CHD. However, a fatigued elderly lady with hypothyroidism and low metabolism might never become physically active enough to stress her heart to the point of developing chest pain, even if she does have CHD. That's what I mean by low thyroid *masking* CHD. For these reasons, doctors are cautious when starting TRT in older people. Initial doses should be lower and upward adjustments slower. The same goes for anyone of any age with known heart problems.

To be clear, appropriate TRT should not be withheld or compromised in the elderly patient; it is simply done more gingerly. At the first sign of worsening cardiac status on TRT, doctors will back off and treat the heart disease. That treatment might involve drugs or revascularization (physically opening the blocked arteries with an angioplasty balloon or bypass surgery). Once the heart problem is stable, adjustment of TRT can be resumed.

But thyroid hormone's effect on the heart is a double-edged sword. That is, heart disease does not always worsen during TRT and it might even improve. The heart's oxygen needs and workload increase as thyroid levels increase, but so does its pumping efficiency. When the heart pumps better, coronary arteries get more blood and cardiac muscle gets more oxygen. So, as long as the increase in oxygen delivery stays ahead of the increase in workload (oxygen need), the patient is better off. When it doesn't, chest pain or a heart attack may strike.

An old Mayo Clinic study looked at fifty-five people with known CHD put on thyroid medication. Nine got worsening chest pain; of those nine, six suffered heart attacks. Now, some people with CHD are going to have a heart attack, so TRT didn't necessarily cause all, or even any, of those attacks. But say it did cause all of them: the worst interpretation of these data is that 16 percent of people (nine out of fifty-five) with CHD worsen on thyroid medicine. That sounds bad, but in twenty-five of the fifty-five people studied, there were no changes in heart status, and twenty-one people actually improved (chest pain completely disappeared in five). So 45 percent didn't change and 38 percent got better. Overall, about 84 percent experienced no worsening of heart disease when starting thyroid hormone. This is all the more remarkable because these cases were collected from the 1930s through the 1950s, when typical doses of thyroid hormone (mostly T_3-containing thyroid USP) were large by today's standards. If the same study were done today, using modern dosing and monitoring, thyroid hormone might come out looking downright heart-friendly.

DURATION OF THYROID REPLACEMENT THERAPY

There are some exceptions, but an individual's need for TRT is usually lifelong. The problems that typically lead to hypothyroidism either don't get better (like a surgically removed thyroid) or cannot be counted upon to do so (like Hashimoto's thyroiditis). In rare cases where there is a reasonable chance of recovery, withdrawal of TRT after a few months can be tried. The problem with doing this routinely is the long half-life of LT_4. It takes five weeks for the drug to clear out of the system and at least a few more weeks for the hypothalamic-pituitary-thyroid (HPT) axis to gear up again. So, it's going to take a couple of months, at least, to see if a patient can fly without TRT. And for some of that time, she'll be enduring hypothyroid symptoms. After all that, if she needs to restart, it'll take another couple of months for levels to build back up. If a patient wants to go through all that, fine. But since TRT is relatively safe, convenient, and cheap, I generally continue it for life unless there is a good reason to do otherwise. One such reason, by the way, would be in a scenario where the patient is given a trial of thyroid pills for suspected hypothyroidism despite normal or borderline lab tests. If reasonable doses for reasonable periods of time don't improve symptoms even a little, then the obvious correct course is to stop the apparently unnecessary treatment before it really does impair internal thyroid system function.

COST OF THYROID REPLACEMENT THERAPY

Thyroid supplements are fairly inexpensive in an era of drugs commonly costing three figures per month. Also, I can't recall having a thyroid prescription rejected for lack of insurance coverage. LT_4 in some form is almost always paid for when patients have prescription drug coverage. In other words, all these drugs are user-friendly, financially and administratively.

I checked an online pharmacy for pricing information on ninety-day supplies of Synthroid, Levoxyl, and generic levothyroxine (100 mcg strength). Synthroid was $35.97, Levoxyl $24.97, and the generic version was $25.97. (Of course, in the news recently, we've been hearing about very-low-cost generics of $4 per month, or $12 for ninety days, being sold by large chains like Wal-Mart.) A roughly equivalent dose of Armour Thyroid (120 mg) runs $25.98 for 90 tablets. Cytomel (LT_3) is $79.98 for 100 tablets (25 mcg). The combined cost for three months of Synthroid 100 mcg plus Cytomel 12.5 mcg (the T_4/T_3 cocktail) would be $71.96, about three times the cost of thyroid USP. Prices, obviously, will vary depending on your location and the source.

Most of these prices are roughly comparable, by the way, to the copayments that insurers commonly require their clients make to get prescriptions filled. In some cases, they might even be cheaper. Don't hesitate, therefore, to ask your pharmacist what your out-of-pocket cost would be to buy your thyroid hormone pills without going through your insurance carrier. We've gotten so used to having most medical costs covered, we almost never consider voluntarily leaving the third-party payer out of the loop..

What are the advantages of doing so? If you can get your thyroid prescription for about the same as what the copay would have been, you'll save your insurance carrier money. If it's a private insurer, maybe your premiums won't go up as much the next year. If it's the government, you can save taxpayers some money. Additionally, if your carrier will not cover anything but generic LT_4, and you and your doctor want Synthroid or the like, then paying out of pocket, if you can afford it, gives you that choice.

CHAPTER 8

MONITORING AND TROUBLESHOOTING THYROID REPLACEMENT

Assessment of hypothyroidism treatment, like its diagnosis, is largely dependent on blood tests, the very same tests we've been discussing. And as with diagnosis, laboratories can be fooled and clinical evaluation is always critical but often ignored. The biochemical goal of thyroid replacement therapy (TRT) is a "normal" thyrotropin (TSH). That means a doctor who calls a TSH level of 4.0 milliunits per liter (mU/L) normal, because the laboratory says it is, probably will be satisfied with a levothyroxine (LT$_4$) dose that results in a TSH of 4.0 mU/L.

TSH TESTING

For all the reasons previously discussed, I believe the target TSH level in thyroid replacement should be no higher than 2.0 or 2.5 mU/L. After all, if TSH levels in the upper half of the reference range represent a mild low-thyroid state for *diagnostic* purposes, then any LT$_4$ dose that results in such a level is mildly inadequate for *therapeutic* purposes. In fact, I consider this factor more critical when monitoring therapy than when trying to make a diagnosis.

What I mean by that is, I have no problem with a doctor saying: "I recognize a TSH higher than 2.0 mU/L is at least borderline abnormal, but I want to wait and see. I'm uncomfortable committing my patient to lifelong treatment until I'm more certain that the problem is going to persist or worsen." Fine. That doctor understands hypothyroidism and is simply being prudent and conservative. What I do have a problem with is committing someone to lifelong therapy, and all the tests and office visits and costs that go with it, and then not making the most of it. I might, for example, hold off treating until I see the TSH level climb above 4.0 mU/L, but once I do start, I'm sure going to get that level below 2.0 mU/L.

The American Association of Clinical Endocrinologists guidelines agree with me in principle, if not in the exact numbers. They don't recommend starting thyroid therapy unless the TSH level is greater than 5.0 mU/L, but their target for therapy is a TSH less than 3.0 mU/L.

Just as in diagnosis, TSH is the best single test for adequacy of TRT. It is often a mistake, however, to rely too heavily on any one test. For that reason, especially in the early stages of TRT, I check a free thyroxine (FT_4) level along with the TSH. The goal is to get the FT_4 somewhere within its reference range, as specified on the laboratory report. In many cases, though, the patient feels best if the FT_4 is run in the upper half of that normal range, just as they do best with a TSH level in the lower half of the normal range. Free triiodothyronine (FT_3) levels are useful less often, but I sometimes get them, especially if I have reason to doubt the reliability of the TSH test. If the TSH is known to be inaccurate, as in central hypothyroidism, I shoot for an FT_4 level in the mid to upper normal range and an FT_3 level somewhere in its normal range.

The Problem of Low TSH

Most of the time, at least in standard practice, a TSH level below the lab's lower normal limit (usually around 0.3 mU/L) indicates the patient's thyroid replacement dose is too high. Generally speaking, dosages should be adjusted to keep TSH levels above that lower limit. There are situations, as foregoing chapters have made clear, where pathological conditions impair the pituitary gland's TSH production and make TSH levels run misleadingly low. We will discuss those on page 133. What I want to discuss here is the significance of low TSH levels in patients whose hypothalamic-pituitary-thyroid (HPT) axis is normal, patients fully capable of generating blood TSH levels appropriate for their blood levels of thyroid hormone.

Physiologically, TSH produced by the pituitary gland travels to the thyroid gland and triggers thyroid hormone production and release. Thyroid hormone, in turn, suppresses further TSH release so hyperthyroidism doesn't develop. In the hypothyroid patient taking levothyroxine (LT$_4$), the same thing happens—T$_4$ from the drug suppresses TSH release by the pituitary. The lower the measured TSH level, the more T$_4$ from the thyroid pill has reached the patient's blood and tissues. The usual practice is to adjust the TRT dose so that the TSH level in a low-thyroid patient is "normal" (by my definition, between about 0.3 and 2.0 mU/L). In other words, doctors generally try to achieve TSHs that are equivalent to those of normal healthy people—people whose thyroid levels are completely under the control of their own HPT axes.

In the TRT patient, mildly low TSH levels worry me a little, but not too much. They might indicate the patient is getting a little more than ideal thyroid hormone, but if the pituitary is still producing some TSH, it's probably not at a dangerously high level. What raises red flags for doctors, me included, is the very low TSH—say, below 0.1 mU/L—and especially the "undetectable" TSH, of less than 0.01 or in some labs, as low as 0.001 mU/L. In this situation, the patient's pituitary gland is getting so much thyroid hormone that it makes little or no TSH. When that happens, the average physician prescribing TRT panics. The LT$_4$ dose is lowered—maybe a little, maybe a lot. And he keeps lowering it more and more, regardless of any other blood levels or patient complaints, until the TSH level increases. The average endocrinologist probably won't panic, but the result is the same. The TRT dose is lowered to keep the TSH level between approximately 0.3 and 2.0 mU/L (or 4.0 mU/L, or whatever, depending on the goal the individual doctor has in mind).

There is a pervasive fear of undetectable or barely detectable TSH levels, and justifiably so. Almost all dangerous—even life-threatening—hyperthyroidism is signaled by a very low TSH. But do all very low TSHs signal dangerous hyperthyroidism? More on that in a moment.

These concerns are not theoretical. Low TSH levels have been conclusively linked with health risks. In one classic study, researchers showed that elderly subjects who had TSH levels that were less than 0.1 mU/L, and normal T_4 levels, were at threefold higher risk of atrial fibrillation, a dangerous form of rapid heartbeat. Now, I'm really splitting hairs here, but the group with TSH levels of less than 0.1 mU/L no doubt included some people with TSHs only slightly less than 0.1—say, 0.08 mU/L—as well as people with significantly higher thyroid levels whose TSHs were far less than 0.1, say, 0.001 mU/L. A TSH level of 0.001 usually will be associated with serious hyperthyroidism, but a TSH of 0.08 might not be. A patient with a TSH of 0.08 might have truly normal or only slightly elevated T_4 and T_3 levels. So, were those in the above-referenced study with TSH levels of around 0.08 mU/L at the same threefold risk of heart rhythm disturbance as the ones with the TSH levels of less than 0.001 mU/L? I don't know, but I bet not.

Here's what I'm getting at. Albert Einstein was famous for his "thought experiments," mainly because his theories were so esoteric for his day that there were few real-world ways to test them. I'm not Albert Einstein, but here's my thought experiment on low TSH levels in thyroid-replacement patients.

In normal people, TSH levels run from 0.3 to 2.0 mU/L or higher. Those levels are needed to trigger production and release of thyroid hormone and to constantly stimulate the thyroid gland, keeping the machinery well-oiled and running. None of that has to happen in a patient on full replacement TRT. Why then should the pituitary bother to make any TSH in a person on just the right dose of LT_4? No reason I can think of. If doctors adjust doses to keep TSH levels in patients comparable to normal people, it might really be running them low. Just barely low, but enough that the pituitary gland keeps doing a little work to help out. In many patients, this postulated deficit is too mild to notice, or their thyroid is able to make up the difference. Others do notice and complain, and doctors ignore them because their TSH levels are normal.

I think this—perhaps more than the whole T_3 question—is why some patients on thyroid hormone pills don't feel right. Perhaps doctors should elevate LT_4 doses enough to just barely make the TSH undetectable or nearly so, to the point that the patient's pituitary senses that no action is needed to augment thyroid hormone sufficiency. Might that be the best means of determining an individual's ideal dose, the point at which the TSH just becomes undetectable? Maybe, but nobody is doing that. I don't think anybody is even asking the question—they're just getting apoplectic over low TSH levels.

If I'm right, and TRT dosing that results in very low TSH levels could be done safely, the process would still not be without risk. Overdosing would be difficult to detect and avoid, so it would be critical to closely monitor T_4 and T_3 levels in addition to symptoms, all of which is time-consuming and expensive. This strategy is beyond the interest and skill levels of many physicians. Endocrinologists could do it in a selected group of patients, but I doubt many would—this course would be even more aggressive than my present practices.

Running TSH levels deliberately low is likely to always be a tough sell. It is a frank violation of the standard of care in 2006. Still, there may be some patients not served well by usual practices who might benefit from careful implementation of this maverick approach.

TESTING FREQUENCY

Frequency of monitoring is one of the sticky wickets in low-thyroid management. LT_4 has a half-life of about a week, and any drug requires five half-lives to reach the condition known as *steady state*. A drug in steady state means that entry of the drug into the bloodstream exactly matches its removal. In other words, the same amount of drug is coming in from the digestive tract (in the case of a drug taken orally) as is going out through drug breakdown and urinary excretion so that blood levels remain constant as long as the drug is taken regularly and reliably. A drug with a short half-life of an hour or two, like amoxicillin, will reach steady state in five to ten hours. LT_4 takes five weeks to reach steady state. This means for a full five weeks after starting LT_4, the serum free thyroxine (FT_4) levels will continue to gradually climb as TSH gradually falls.

It is usually unnecessary to do any testing or make any dose adjustments prior to five weeks, and to do so may be counterproductive. It is essential for patients to understand this, so they don't expect results too quickly. I tell patients they will probably start feeling better in a week, but it could be a month or two before the full effect of TRT is felt.

In addition to waiting for a steady state to be reached, one needs to allow for the rather plodding pace of many of the effects of thyroid hormone. Triiodothyronine (T_3) binds its receptor and triggers DNA transcription into RNA, and RNA translation into new proteins. Levels of these proteins need time to build in order to produce their effects. How long does all this take? It's different for every tissue and for each of the many effects of thyroid hormone. Over and above the five weeks it takes blood levels of T_4 to build up, I tend to tack on at least a week, perhaps a month, before I really expect a patient to feel better.

How long a doctor waits before retesting after a dose change is a good litmus test for how competent he or she is with thyroid disease. Except in unusual circumstances, less than five or six weeks is too soon, and greater than three or four months is too long. Pregnancy is one of those unusual circumstances, by the way. Because normal thyroid hormone levels are critical to fetal development, and because hormone requirements increase as pregnancy progresses, I generally retest two to four weeks after a dose change just to be sure things are moving in the right direction.

FULL REPLACEMENT OR LESS?

If the goals of TRT are met on a particular dose of thyroid medication—the test results look good, the patient feels well—is it ever necessary to increase the dose further? *Full-replacement dose* is that amount of LT_4 necessary to provide 100 percent of a patient's daily thyroid hormone requirement. That is, TRT has fully replaced her thyroid gland with pills. A patient's full-replacement dose can be estimated mathematically by the following formula:

$$\text{Body weight in pounds} \times 0.72 = LT_4 \text{ dose in micrograms}$$

Roughly equivalent to 75 micrograms (mcg) per 100 pounds of body weight, this equation is generally accepted by the mainstream, but it only gets you in the ballpark. To use myself as an example: I weigh about 130 pounds, so my calculated full-replacement dose is $130 \times 0.72 = 93.6$ mcg. Based on that calculation, I should be taking between 88 mcg and 100 mcg every day. But from long experience, I have found that the dose I need to keep my TSH at a noncontroversial "normal" level is somewhere around 137 or 150 mcg per day. The formula isn't perfect because it doesn't account for activity, physical conditioning, interfering drugs, body fat percentages, and so forth. But it is a useful gauge for determining if patients are greatly overdosed or underdosed relative to full-replacement needs. This can be helpful in situations like central hypothyroidism, where TSH levels aren't reliable and doctors need additional clues to make good decisions about dosing TRT.

Do we need to fully replace if, as in some people, the goals of TRT can be achieved at a lesser dose? That is, if the patient's own thyroid gland is decent enough to make up the difference? I usually do give full replacement even if the deficiency is mild, but I'm pretty aggressive in my treatment strategy. Not everyone would agree with that, which is fine.

Here is an example, however, illustrating the potential disadvantage of not providing full replacement. Say that Andrea needs 100 mcg of T_4 to get through the day. If her own thyroid gland manages to wring out 75 mcg per day, then a small LT_4 dose of 25 mcg will do the trick, right? Probably. What if by six months later her Hashimoto's thyroiditis has wreaked more havoc on her thyroid system to the point where she can only manufacture 50 mcg per day. Andrea will be short 25 mcg per day again, despite our efforts. If her follow-up appointment with me is still months off, and she doesn't call to let me know there's a problem, she spends that time living with the same symptoms she had before. (Don't let this happen—keep your doctor informed.) Eventually, Andrea decides LT_4 doesn't work or her doctor isn't skilled enough to handle her condition. I've had plenty of people discontinue their hormone pills in this situation. Honestly, I think a lot of the frustration from patients and a lot of the condemnation of mainstream doctors' hypothyroidism care stem from this very scenario: well-meaning, reasonable, *partial* replacement.

In the above example, partial replacement was suboptimal because an initial improvement was quickly lost, leaving the patient in the same situation she had been in before treatment. Here's another, slightly different possibility to consider. Less than full-replacement dose TRT might make things worse rather than better, or even the same. This is speculation, but let me illustrate with a nonhormonal example.

Doctors are taught in medical school never to give partial antibiotic treatment for an infection. With partial treatment, the most susceptible (say 80 percent) of bacteria die quickly. The remaining 20 percent of the germ population, which is mildly drug-resistant and would have been killed by a higher dose or a longer course of antibiotics, survive to reproduce. With no competition from the 80 percent of bugs that are now dead, the offspring of the 20 percent grow faster and hardier than they otherwise would have. Also, the average bacterium is more antibiotic-resistant than it was at the beginning. A second treatment will be less effective than the first, so the doctor has made the situation worse by providing partial therapy. Better to hit an infection with high doses for an extended period from the outset.

Is there a thyroid analogy to the development of antibiotic resistance? Let's say Andrea's struggling thyroid was just barely able to squeeze out that 75 mcg per day it was producing before TRT. Once it perceives that help is on the way in the form of a Levoxyl tablet, it might relax a little. The 25 mcg arrives from outside and suddenly Andrea's thyroid only makes 65 mcg a day, leaving her with a total of 90 mcg to work with, or 10 mcg short of what she needs.

With this in mind, I might treat Andrea with 100 mcg (her full-replacement dose) from the outset. But what about that 75 mcg she is making—won't it combine with the 100 mcg she swallows and make her hyperthyroid with 175 mcg per day? Not as long as her hypothalamic-pituitary-thyroid (HPT) axis functions correctly (no hormone resistance, for example, mucking up the works). As soon as the central part of Andrea's thyroid system detects more than 100 mcg of T_4 in a day, thyrotropin-releasing hormone (TRH) and thyrotropin (TSH) levels will both fall to prevent prolonged thyroid excess. This is called down-regulation of the HPT axis.

Some patients treated as I have just described complain of jitteriness and other hyperthyroid symptoms during the first week, which later resolve. I suspect this represents a delay between the rise in thyroid levels from outside and internal down-regulation. This is rarely a problem, especially if thyroid levels were pretty low to begin with. But if the starting levels are close to normal, or if the patient is elderly or has heart disease, I sometimes recommend taking half the ordered dose for the first week or two. In other words, ease into full replacement.

WHEN GOOD LABS LIE

Just as in the diagnostic phase of hypothyroidism management, situations arise in treatment where TSH levels inaccurately reflect the correctness of a dose of LT_4. Obviously, in central hypothyroidism, TSH testing is unreliable, and it probably shouldn't even be done. If it is, the result will be lower than expected for any given level of free thyroxine (FT_4). And though TSH production from the pituitary gland won't go up as it should when thyroid levels fall, TSH falls just fine when thyroid levels rise. For this reason, undetectable TSH levels commonly result from properly treated central hypothyroidism. Underdosing of LT_4 may occur, though, when the unwary doctor tries in vain to get this low TSH up to "normal" by giving less and less drug. I see this happen frequently, because many primary-care doctors do not know how to treat central hypothyroidism.

In most cases of thyroid hormone resistance, TSH runs higher than expected relative to FT_4 and FT_3. Whether or not the LT_4 dose should be increased to get the TSH level down depends on whether the central and peripheral ends of the system are in balance. Clearly, evaluation for signs and symptoms of both hyper- and hypothyroidism is critical in people on TRT, especially if the TSH level is suspect. In treatment, just as with diagnosis, neither lab tests nor the clinical situation should ever be contemplated in isolation.

THYROID REPLACEMENT AFTER HYPERTHYROIDISM

Because it is such a common situation, I want to make special mention of the patient on TRT following the correction of high thyroid levels. Most often, these people have had Graves' disease treated with radioactive iodine to destroy part of the thyroid gland. Largely, the hypothyroidism in these patients is handled just like everybody else's, but three things are different: weight problems, post-hyperthyroid central hypothyroidism, and persistent thyroid-stimulating immunoglobulins (TSIs).

Weight

Graves' disease (the most common internal cause of hyperthyroidism) often causes weight loss. Once treated, the patient frequently expresses shock and distress over rapid weight gain. These pounds come from three sources: (1) desirable restoration of weight lost due to the illness, (2) potential weight gain caused by post-treatment primary hypothyroidism, and (3) lack of exercise and excess calorie intake carried over from the hyperthyroid state (that is, the patient got used to being able to eat more and exercise less without gaining weight in the midst of the hypermetabolism of Graves' disease). I mention all of this to point out that weight may be a bigger problem in this category of hypothyroidism than others. Frustration is common and attention to diet, exercise, and precise thyroid hormone dosing is critical.

Post-Hyperthyroid Central Hypothyroidism

Post-hyperthyroid central hypothyroidism (PHCH) is my designation for leftover HPT axis suppression following thyroid hormone excess. This almost always happens in the few weeks to months after hyperthyroid treatment. The TSH test should never be trusted to guide dose adjustments during this time. In some cases, PHCH may persist, with the thyroid gas gauge stuck on "F." I always question the reliability of TSH levels in the post-hyperthyroid patient, even if she had Graves' disease treated decades ago. If I can find in her records, though, that her TSH level rose very high at some point—greater than, say, 50 mU/L—then PHCH probably isn't present.

Persistent TSIs

In Graves' disease, antibodies called thyroid-stimulating immunoglobulins (TSIs) cause the thyroid to overact. TSIs sometimes remain after the thyroid has been destroyed by radioactive iodine and act like poltergeists, sneaking around unseen and causing lots of mischief.

In the successfully treated Graves' disease patient, who is now hypothyroid on TRT, persistent TSIs may cause low TSH levels in two ways: by ultra-short-loop feedback or by stimulation of residual thyroid tissue. In the former, the patient may be clinically normal and adjustment of the LT_4 dose may not be needed. In the latter, the patient is truly hyperthyroid (over-replaced) and the thyroid hormone dose should be lowered.

Ultra-short-loop feedback is a recently discovered nuance of HPT axis function in normal people. Basically, this means that some TSH released from the pituitary gland routinely does a U-turn and binds to receptors on the pituitary itself, helping to shut off further TSH production. In a post-treatment Graves' disease patient, TSIs can bind to these same receptors and lower TSH levels without any help at all from the TRT hormone pill. This isn't a problem as long as the doctor realizes the TSH is not accurately reflecting the patient's thyroid status. Just as in central hypothyroidism, TRT doses in this situation should be adjusted according to signs and symptoms, and FT_4 and FT_3 levels.

The other way that persisting TSIs might lower TSH levels in a treated Graves' disease patient involves residual surviving thyroid tissue. When I said that radioactive iodine destroys the thyroid gland, I was oversimplifying—some thyroid tissue always survives. If it's only a little and TSI levels are low, no problem. But if TSIs stay high and there are enough surviving thyroid follicular cells, internal thyroid hormone production that isn't inhibited by LT_4 continues.

Let me clarify what I am proposing. Diane needs 100 mcg of T_4 a day. While she has Graves' disease, she makes 200 mcg. She gets treated with radioactive iodine and now makes 50 mcg, half of which is under the control of TSIs (Graves' disease) and half under normal HPT axis control. I give her full-replacement LT_4, 100 mcg per day. The portion of her internal production under HPT axis control gets suppressed as usual, but the 25 mcg under TSI control doesn't budge. On TRT, therefore, she ends up with 125 mcg T_4 per day—100 mcg from outside and 25 mcg from inside.

I can tell from routine tests that she's hyperthyroid, but not why. I decrease her LT_4 to 75 mcg. That amount plus the 25 produced internally gives her 100 mcg. Normal, and everybody's happy.

That is until TSI levels fluctuate up or down, which they do unpredictably. This needs to be considered in a Graves' disease patient after radioactive iodine treatment, if the patient's TRT requirements go up and down a lot for no apparent reason. A blood test for TSIs will confirm what's happening. The cure is another radioactive iodine dose to get rid of the surviving thyroid tissue.

Ultra-short-loop feedback has been shown to occur in peer-reviewed research, while TSI stimulation of residual thyroid tissue, to my knowledge, has not been. On the other hand, I am proposing in the latter scenario nothing more than the notion that sometimes a single dose of radioactive iodine does not completely cure the hyperthyroidism of Graves' disease—an undisputed fact. And regardless of the details, the bottom line is that TSH is not a reliable guide to adjusting TRT in patients with high post-treatment TSI levels. Doctors should take great care to assure that the Graves' disease patient is truly over-replaced before dropping her dose of TRT.

ADVERSE EFFECTS OF THYROID REPLACEMENT

Logically, levothyroxine (LT_4) should be free of side effects. It is chemically identical to the major natural product of the thyroid gland, so patients are getting nothing that normal humans don't make for themselves every day. Except, of course, for the food coloring and other ingredients mingled inside the hormone pill, which, rarely, can cause allergic reactions. We get around that when necessary by using 50 microgram (mcg) tablets, which are white and contain no dyes.

Now, I'd be the first to raise an eyebrow at anybody declaring any drug, even LT_4, to be absolutely without adverse effects. This is not a risk-free world. A pharmacology professor of mine once said, "All drugs are poisons." But as medications go, LT_4 is pretty clean, provided it's not overdosed. In people who aren't overdosed and don't have allergies to food coloring, LT_4 shouldn't cause side effects. Obviously, though, dose adjustments involve trial and error, which can result in transient mild overdosing and underdosing—and, hence, hypothyroidism and hyperthyroidism—in almost everybody at one time or another.

Overdosing

The adverse consequences of excessive thyroid replacement therapy include the direct effects of too much thyroid hormone on the body and, potentially, long-term suppression of the hypothalamic-pituitary-thyroid (HPT) axis.

Hyperthyroidism

If overdosed, the TRT patient becomes hyperthyroid. Some symptoms of high thyroid, any or all of which could result from too much LT_4, include the following:

- Nervousness, hand tremors, restlessness, irritability

- Insomnia

- Fatigue

- Heat intolerance, sweating

- Weight loss

- Rapid or irregular heartbeat

- Frequent bowel movements

- Muscle weakness

- Depression

HPT Axis Suppression

Just as internally driven hyperthyroidism can suppress brain and pituitary gland control of the thyroid system, so can externally (that is, hormone pill) derived high thyroid. As long as TRT is continued, particularly if at or near the full-replacement dose, this shouldn't be a problem. In the rare iﬂstance that a patient might be able to stop therapy, however, past over-dosing of LT_4 may temporarily, if not permanently, prevent her own system from functioning normally again. In other words, excessive TRT can cause post-hyperthyroid central hypothyroidism (PHCH).

Theoretically, this shouldn't happen as long as TSH levels stay above the laboratory's lower limit of normal, generally around 0.3 mU/L. Persistence of a normal TSH level is a simple indicator that the HPT axis is still operating. But I worry that full-replacement doses (such as I recommend) or any accidental or deliberate treatment that runs the TSH frankly low, may lessen the ability of the HPT axis to completely and rapidly retake control if ever called upon to do so.

This is a well-known problem with the adrenal system—why not with the thyroid? Yet, doctors give this possible consequence of TRT remarkably little attention. PHCH, by the way, is an excellent reason to avoid undetectable TSH levels during TRT. Ignoring the potential risks of too much thyroid hormone, as is done by some reformists advocating T_3-only therapy, could wreck the HPT axis and the person's ability to ever make thyroid hormone naturally again. My own earlier proposal about escalating therapy just to the point that the TSH becomes undetectable (see pages 126–129) should only be considered if more standard therapy fails, and such therapy must be carried out very carefully. At this point, I would add that it should only be done in cases where there is no chance of the patient ever coming off of TRT, and so no chance of the patient ever needing a functioning HPT axis again. One example of such a situation would be complete surgical removal of the thyroid.

Unmasking

In addition to the direct adverse effects of TRT just discussed, some patients complain of problems unrelated to a true drug side effect, which are nevertheless perceived to be triggered by thyroid hormone pills. And in a sense they are, indirectly. I call this set of problems "unmasking."

The desired effect of LT_4 in a hypothyroid patient is to awaken the body, metabolically speaking. The brain becomes more alert and active, the heart beats harder, and blood vessels open up to accommodate a more vigorous circulation. Patients may feel more energetic and less depressed and hence increase their physical activity. All this sounds great, if the only problem is hypothyroidism. But low thyroid can mask other conditions; in other words, the treatment of low thyroid might aggravate other conditions.

Perhaps the newly alert brain takes sudden notice of a nagging problem lurking in the shadows. Or the hypothyroid symptoms, now gone, may have been severe enough to distract the brain from these other discomforts. Either way, TRT makes the person more aware of symptoms that might have nothing to do with too much or too little thyroid hormone. These—not new, but *newly perceived*—complaints may be blamed on LT_4 or mistaken for features of hypothyroidism not responding to therapy. In other words, the new complaint might be interpreted as either a side effect or a failure of TRT, when it is in fact neither.

We previously discussed an important example of unmasking: TRT's potential exacerbation of heart disease. Taking Synthroid will not cause artery blockages leading to angina and heart attacks (if anything, it helps prevent them), but the correction of hypothyroidism can destabilize existing heart disease. TRT stimulates the metabolism and need for oxygen in all tissues, including the heart. In addition, the treated low-thyroid patient may feel suddenly better than she has in years: she may jog or clean the whole house or go on an adventurous vacation, when a month before she didn't feel like crawling out of bed. A sick heart might be unable to adjust quickly to the increased exertion, leading to a myocardial infarction. Did LT_4 cause her heart attack? Only indirectly. LT_4 corrected a problem that was keeping her heart disease in check, but the heart disease was there like a wolf in the fold, caused by genes, years of poor diet and lack of exercise, maybe smoking or diabetes, and perhaps the hypothyroidism itself. But it wasn't caused by LT_4.

I've seen properly prescribed LT_4 seemingly trigger epilepsy, anxiety attacks, migraine headaches, and bipolar depression. My patients already had these disorders, which were masked (hidden) by the decreased metabolism of hypothyroidism. When LT_4 stripped that mask away and metabolism rose again, the original problems returned. Not an *adverse* effect of LT_4, but a *beneficial* effect of low thyroid removed. It's a subtle distinction and I've had patients refuse to accept it. As a result, they might refuse to take TRT in proper doses or at all. The answer is not to leave hypothyroidism untreated, however, but to have the other condition treated aggressively before, or simultaneously with, the thyroid condition.

Poor musculoskeletal and cardiovascular conditioning may also be unmasked by thyroid replacement. A person fatigued by hypothyroidism may have been inactive for months or years, resulting in poor physical fitness. "Use it or lose it." She didn't use it, perhaps because of hypothyroidism, but she lost it because of how Mother Nature made us—her heart, muscles, and even skeleton grew weak from lack of exercise.

Take Irene, for example, a woman with years of underactivity behind her due to hypothyroidism. She takes LT_4. Time passes and her lab tests are perfect. She feels great and exerts herself. Her muscles get sore when they get worked more than they're used to. That's normal—"no pain, no gain." Her weak joints ache too, and because of poor cardiovascular fitness, she becomes short-winded and exhausted from the least activity. She's no longer feeling better. By the time she sees me again in the office, she complains of just as much fatigue and achiness as before. "These pills just aren't working," she moans.

Patients have often told me they initially felt better after starting TRT, then the symptoms crept back. Is this new pain and fatigue caused by hypothyroidism not improving because LT_4 therapy is not working, or are they normal consequences of prolonged inactivity, which no amount of thyroid hormone will ever fix? I think this last scenario might be a common one.

TROUBLESHOOTING THYROID REPLACEMENT

Many people on TRT, myself included, do quite well. In those who do not—those who perceive ineffectiveness or side effects from their thyroid medication—multiple possible reasons exist. The following are potential problems and their solutions.

POTENTIAL PROBLEM	SOLUTION
1. Complaint wholly unrelated to the thyroid problem	Diagnose and treat the complaint
2. Inadequate implementation of TRT	Implement solution specified below
a. TSH allowed to remain greater than 2.0–2.5 mU/L	Increase the LT_4 dose
b. Failure to add LT_3 to LT_4 in cases where it is needed	Add Cytomel (LT_3)
c. Failure to push the dose upward to at or near the calculated full-replacement dose	Increase the LT_4 dose
3. Unmasking of a nonthyroidal problem previously made better or less noticeable by hypothyroidism	Implement solution specified below
a. Exacerbation of an existing condition (for example, new or worsening angina in a person with underlying coronary heart disease)	Treat the condition
b. Poor physical or cardiovascular conditioning	Start a gradually escalating exercise program

Part of the art and science of managing hypothyroidism is figuring out what's wrong at times when all is not well. Is the problem with the medicine or how it is given? Or is the problem within the patient? How do I convince myself and a suffering patient that the medication is fine? The solution to her problem might be, for example, a difficult lifestyle change, perhaps deliberate infliction of more discomfort (exercise, for instance) before things get better. Normal tests do part of the convincing, but time and again we've seen that tests don't tell the whole story. Some trial-and-error changes in TRT dose, maybe even trying LT_3, are reasonable. But if altering the TRT dose doesn't seem to make much difference, the solution probably lies elsewhere.

RECIPE FOR SUCCESS

The following is my protocol for starting thyroid replacement therapy (TRT), adjusting the dose, and monitoring the patient's response in presumed *primary* hypothyroidism. Management of central hypothyroidism is similar, but thyrotropin (TSH) testing is always unreliable. This outline summarizes everything we've discussed so far. You may wish to go over it with your doctor if your TRT doesn't seem to be going as planned.

All LT_4 dosage adjustments, up or down, are generally made in 12.5 mcg to 25 mcg increments. Unless specified, the patient is assumed to be under fifty years of age, with no heart disease. If you are over fifty and/or have heart disease, the same principles apply, but more caution is needed.

Starting Therapy

To begin thyroid replacement therapy:

1. Take a branded LT_4 (Synthroid, Levoxyl, Levothroid, or Unithroid) and generally stick with that brand for the duration.

2. Start with 50–100 mcg per day or about 0.72 mcg per pound of body weight per day (roughly 75 mcg per 100 pounds), whichever is least.

    a. Underdosing is better than overdosing at this stage.

    b. In older patients, especially those with heart disease, I start with no more than 12.5 mcg to 25 mcg per day.

    c. If the hypothyroidism is very mild (say, a TSH level only slightly higher than 2.0 mU/L), then I follow the same guidelines, but instruct the patient to take half the ordered pill for the first one to two weeks to prevent transient hyperthyroidism.

Monitoring and Adjusting Therapy

Once on TRT it is important to evaluate the results, and act accordingly. I do so as follows:

1. Check the TSH and free thyroxine (FT_4) levels no sooner than five weeks and no longer than about twelve weeks after starting TRT.

    a. If the TSH level is high (greater than 2.0 mU/L, generally), then I increase the LT_4 dose.

b. If the TSH level is low (less than 0.3 mU/L, generally), then I look at the FT_4 level.

(1) If the FT_4 level is normal (using the laboratory's reference range), then I generally decrease the LT_4 dose; however, if the TSH is only mildly low and the patient is doing well clinically, I would consider making no change.

(2) If the FT_4 level is high, then I decrease the LT_4 dose.

(3) If the FT_4 level is low, then central hypothyroidism is possible and I increase the LT_4 dose with a goal of getting the FT_4 level into the upper half of the normal range (careful observation for high-thyroid symptoms is required in case the TSH test is accurate and the FT_4 turns out to be in error).

c. If the TSH level is normal, then I evaluate signs, symptoms, and the FT_4 level carefully.

(1) If the FT_4 level is normal and the patient has no clinical evidence of hypothyroidism, then I make no change.

(2) If the FT_4 level is normal but the patient remains clinically hypothyroid, then:

- A small increase in LT_4 dose might result in an FT_4 level a little higher within the goal range and a TSH level a little lower in the goal range, with better symptom control.

- Thyroid hormone resistance is possible, in which case a small increase in LT_4 dose is still reasonable.

(3) A high FT_4 level raises several possibilities:

- The combination of normal TSH level, high FT_4 level, plus clinical hypothyroidism (or perhaps even hyperthyroidism) is most often caused by the patient skipping LT_4 doses (causing a rise in TSH), then overdosing in the week or so prior to testing (causing the rise in FT_4) to hide her failure to follow directions. (Which never happens, right?)

- If the patient feels fine, then the high FT_4 level may indicate peripheral thyroid hormone resistance, where more LT_4 than usual is required to treat symptoms and normalize TSH. Sometimes FT_4 levels just run high in the early stages of TRT and will decline later. Either way, I would not change the LT_4 dose.

- If the patient is clinically hyperthyroid, then the LT_4 dose probably should be lowered.

(4) If the FT_4 level is low:

- If the patient feels fine, then I either change nothing or cautiously increase the LT_4 dose.
- If the patient is clinically hypothyroid, then there is probably a defect in TSH production (central hypothyroidism) and I increase the LT_4 dose.

2. Whenever the LT_4 dose is changed, I check TSH and FT_4 levels in six to twelve weeks and repeat the above analysis.

Follow-up

Further actions depend on how everything has gone previously:

1. If a hormone dose is found that yields a clinically normal patient and acceptable test numbers, then I recheck the TSH (FT_4 is optional at this stage if the TSH test is deemed reliable) in six months (sooner, if new complaints arise).

   a. If everything checks out normally at six months, yearly visits are reasonable.

   b. If at any point signs, symptoms, or tests suggest high-thyroid or low-thyroid status, the situation must be re-analyzed.

2. If a reasonable effort (several rounds of adjustment and retesting) finds no LT_4-only dose that clears the bulk of the patient's hypothyroid complaints without making the TSH low, four possibilities exist:

   a. The complaints might be nonthyroid in nature (see discussion on unmasking).

   b. The patient might be on a less than full-replacement dose. If so, I try a gradual increase toward full replacement (estimated at 0.72 mcg per pound body weight per day).

c. The patient could have central hypothyroidism or peripheral resistance to thyroid hormone (the peripheral half of the system more resistant than the central half). Either way (distinguishing the two may be impossible), I ignore the low TSH level and increase the LT_4 dose as high as necessary to get symptom control.

(1) In central hypothyroidism, the FT_4 level should still be a good indicator of thyroid status, and a high FT_4 level should be avoided.

(2) In thyroid hormone resistance, a high FT_4 level is not always inappropriate.

(3) Magnetic resonance imaging (MRI) of the pituitary gland should be considered here, since one cause of central hypothyroidism is a pituitary tumor.

(4) The proposed solution to increase the LT_4 dose as high as necessary does put the patient at risk of dangerous hyperthyroid side effects if the diagnosis is wrong, especially if the TSH is rendered undetectable as opposed to just mildly low. This diagnosis and action should be considered as a last resort, although it is possible that this situation is relatively common but rarely recognized. The patient should be informed of the risks and uncertainties involved. Such nonstandard treatment should only be ordered by a well-qualified physician, usually an endocrinologist.

d. The fourth possibility is defective T_3 hormone production.

(1) Causes include poor T_4 to T_3 peripheral conversion; or lack of direct T_3 hormone secretion from what's left of the patient's thyroid gland, due to near-complete thyroid destruction (by disease, surgery, or radiation) or excessive past or present LT_4 doses suppressing the hypothalamic-pituitary-thyroid axis.

(2) I advise a trial of combined T_4/T_3 therapy at this point.

• I lower the LT_4 dose by 25–50 mcg per day and add LT_3 (Cytomel), 5 mcg twice per day or 12.5 mcg every morning.

- I then retest as above (under the heading "Monitoring and Adjusting Therapy"), but add a FT_3 test to the TSH and FT_4 tests.
- Adjustments are trickier with two drugs, but the goals are the same (a usual TSH level of 0.3–2.0 mU/L, normal FT_4, and FT_3 levels, and no symptoms). It helps to recall that the FT_4 level can only be affected by LT_4, while the FT_3 level is influenced by both LT_3 and LT_4 (the latter via peripheral conversion). That is, adjusting the LT_3 dose will only affect FT_3 levels, but adjusting the LT_4 dose will affect both FT_4 and FT_3. Generally, I leave the LT_3 dose as is and adjust the LT_4 dose up or down as needed.

There it is—my version of the holy grail. You might think it complicated. It is and most doctors would agree. Remember, though, it's dangerous to oversimplify complicated subjects. Fortunately, LT_4-only therapy works fine for most people, and most of the time the test results fall into place. Most hypothyroid patients won't need to venture below the first few lines of my protocol. The ones who do, though, should be seeing an experienced, open-minded specialist to help sort through the complexity of all this. Under no circumstances should a person try to work through this labyrinth on her or his own.

CHAPTER 9

ESCAPING THE PARADOX

Hypothyroidism is a disease known to be common that, paradoxically, may be rampantly overlooked. When I contemplated writing about this paradox of hypothyroidism—the disease we know so well, yet often don't seem to know at all—I assumed the result would be controversial, even heretical, in my professional circle. Not that I sought controversy, but I had things to say about my years of caring for thyroid patients, conclusions and concerns sprouting from those experiences that I thought would be labeled maverick at best, and crackpot at worst, by my mainstream peers. My intent was to present reasonable speculations, extrapolating modern thyroidology into uncharted territory.

To my surprise, though, as I waded into the project, I found published support in widely respected mainstream journals and texts for almost everything I wanted to say. Thus, with the realization that I was coloring less outside the lines than I thought, my approach changed. I became, in my own mind, less a rebel battling hardheaded science, and more a slayer of myths, myths pervading modern thyroidology as it is routinely practiced. These include:

- the myth of the infallible TSH test
- the myth of the unreliability of clinical findings in hypothyroidism
- the myth that levothyroxine is the only therapeutic option and that T_3-containing treatments are obsolete and dangerous
- the myth that weight gain and thyroid problems are not associated

- the myth that complaints resistant to usual thyroid treatment "can't be your thyroid"

The problem, I came to realize, is not a lack of data. There are gaps in our knowledge, but gaps aren't the problem—poor acknowledgement that they exist is. Back in the late 1980s and early 1990s, when I was in training, there was a notion that the thyroid was boring. Nothing new remained to be learned. Clearly, those were false beliefs. How close-minded and conceited—yet many doctors still think that the functioning of the thyroid is as simple as it was taught to them. Which brings us back to *The Thyroid Paradox's* stated purpose: "To correct the pervasive oversimplification of thyroid science and of most of the care given to thyroid patients today."

COOKING SOUFFLÉS IN AN EASY-BAKE OVEN

Doctors have dumbed down hypothyroidism management in a number of fundamental ways:

- By depending almost exclusively on hypothalamic-pituitary-thyroid (HPT) axis testing to assess the entire system
- By thinking that nothing ever breaks other than the thyroid gland (and perhaps once or twice the pituitary gland)
- By trusting laboratory test reports to define "normal"
- By treating numbers, not patients
- By giving only enough thyroid medicine—never a smidgen more—to make the TSH level fall somewhere, *any*where, between two numbers on a piece of paper
- By not listening to patients, whose treatment may be falling short
- By not educating the ones who think thyroid hormone pills will solve every ill, ranging from poor fitness, to soreness from exertion, to the consequences of an overstressed lifestyle

Caring for hypothyroidism is more than just reading a number and writing a prescription (or not writing one). Sometimes it *is* that simple, often it is not. Why this mainstreamist drive toward thyroid simplism? Honest oversights or misapplications of facts partly explain it. Other reasons, though, arise disturbingly out of, I think, misguided social and economic agendas.

I was surprised and a little disquieted to learn that there is a federal government office, called the Agency for Healthcare Research and Quality, a part of whose mandate is the promotion of evidence-based medicine (EBM). They, in part, sponsored a paper I cited earlier proclaiming there to be no justification for doctors to screen patients for thyroid disease. This opinion happens to be in opposition to recommendations of the American College of Physicians and the American Thyroid Association (whose memberships consist of thousands of doctors taking care of millions of patients). EBM, it seems, and in some respects, the United States government, don't want your cryptic thyroid disease to be found. Too much bother, I guess, to unearth those 8 million undiagnosed hypothyroid patients whose existence was inferred by another federal project, the Third National Health and Nutritional Examination Survey (NHANES III), much less the even larger numbers I've conjectured about.

Evidence-based medicine is defined as the "judicious use of the best available evidence from clinical research in making clinical decisions." Not that there's anything wrong with that, on its face. The problem comes with the use of peer-reviewed evidence *alone* to create definitive practice guidelines, which ends up boiling medicine down to the lowest common denominator. It gives us a notion of the way things *usually* are, but *always* and *never* don't exist in medicine. Some patient, somewhere, will break the rules. And doctors trained to excessively focus on evidence are liable to miss problems in those rulebreaking patients and do them a disservice. Practicing EBM indiscriminately, to be blunt, risks delivering substandard care to anybody whose problem doesn't fit the mainstream's current notion of "typical."

Dr. Victor Montori, of the Mayo Clinic, in his previously mentioned paper in *Endocrine Practice*, declared: "Without clinical expertise, a well-intentioned clinical apprentice armed with the best available evidence will likely cause more harm than good." So, one problem with EBM is its failure to account for biological diversity. Another is that the foundation it's built upon is data that may or may not accurately reflect the truth. Are estrogen pills good or bad for the heart? Different decade, different answer. And obviously EBM's value is limited to areas where sufficient quality research has been published. It cannot cover every situation because we don't know everything.

Physicians will always find it necessary to muddle along on incomplete information. I'm afraid, though, the more we train new doctors to suck from the teat of EBM, the less skilled they will be in dealing with diversity and the unknown. Hard data should be exploited when possible, but we mustn't be so starstruck by the 20 percent or 50 percent of something we *do* know that we charge forth, blithely ignoring the 50 percent or 80 percent we *don't*.

EBM and its handmaiden, the clinical practice guideline, are tools that, in skillful hands, provide advice to be accepted or rejected. But good health care must be individualized based on patients' needs and doctors' experiences, perceptions, and instincts. EBM can help, but it must not be used to create an army of Stepford doctors.

WHY EVIDENCE-BASED MEDICINE?

I think three factors have driven the rise of evidence-based medicine and the compulsion to simplify rightfully complex problems: time, knowledge, and cost.

Time

To make ends meet, doctors sometimes see more patients than they can give adequate attention to. Supply and demand, too few doctors in the area to support the patient load, might also drive overbooking. Whatever the cause, less time per patient means less time for thoughtful consideration and serious research into that person's problem. The path of least resistance is to blindly follow mentors, experts, drug company representatives, published articles, and simple guidelines, rather than to think for oneself and question "definitive" sources. It's easily forgotten that questioning is good; it is the first step, after all, in any scientific inquiry.

Knowledge

The more complicated and technical medicine becomes, the greater the legitimate need for doctors to seek expert outside opinions on how to deal with important disorders. Clinical practice guidelines, one source of such opinions, are reasonable and necessary. Doctors must simply make sure that one author's or group's recommended way of doing something isn't mistaken for the *only* way, always and forever.

Cost

Medical care is expensive. The more uniform everybody's care becomes, however, the cheaper it gets. If a hospital knows how many pneumonia patients to expect, and knows each will be treated with antibiotic X because that's what the guidelines say, then they can buy antibiotic X in bulk and save money. That's not necessarily bad, but will there be room in the budget for a doctor wishing to exercise his or her free choice and prescribe antibiotic Y or Z instead?

Lack of free choice for the doctor and patient within the typically broad range of acceptable options in health care is problematic in and of itself. It's especially so if the person figuring out which option to mandate is a third party—a third party who's footing the bill. That's what is happening when the government or some other insurer gets in the act. It's happening, for example, every time you're told that the drug you've just been prescribed isn't on your insurance carrier's formulary. Cost containment must be a concern, but it should never be the overriding one.

Physician Extenders

A method commonly used by doctors to manage two of the above problems is to employ physician extenders (PEs)—that is, nurse practitioners or physician's assistants. According to the *New England Journal of Medicine*, 36 percent of Americans get care from these nonphysicians. PEs address the time factor by helping the office see more patients, while presumably still giving each one adequate face-to-face attention. That lowers cost because a PE isn't paid as much as a fully credentialed physician. But are they as well trained or as broadly experienced?

Without intending to insult any hardworking, dedicated, highly qualified people, there are obvious differences between physicians and PEs that might affect the quality of patient care delivered, analogous to similar differences between specialist and generalist physicians. Compared to the average doctor, PEs are probably more frequently going to run into clinical situations where they are unsure how to proceed. That's not a crippling problem because PEs can ask for help, provided the individual recognizes and acts appropriately when his or her level of competence is being exceeded. That's the way the arrangement is supposed to work: a PE is supposed to be supervised by a physician who reviews the PE's cases and is available to answer questions. In my experience and opinion, some PEs are well supervised, and some aren't.

But evidence-based medicine swoops down to save the day. When a collection of simplified step-by-step instructions—a "cookbook"—is employed for dealing with complicated diseases, then PEs can do more without expensive supervision. EBM allows extenders to work cheaper and faster, and hands them free rein in more situations, perhaps fostering a false sense of competence when the PE might really be in too deep.

With evidence-based medicine, more of your health care can be done by nonphysicians. Much of the time, that's okay. Particularly in roles where there is a well-defined, limited scope of care, PEs function superbly, an example being nurse practitioners working with diabetic patients—providing education, insulin-pump starts, adjustments of a limited assortment of medications, and so on. But when it comes to thinking outside the box—violating the cookbook, for example, by considering prescribing thyroid replacement for a clinically hypothyroid patient with normal lab tests—extenders are not as well equipped, especially considering that primary-care physicians and endocrinologists make plenty of thyroid mistakes all by themselves.

YOU CAN ESCAPE THE PARADOX

Complex medical issues are being simplified by excessive reliance on clinical practice guidelines and peer-reviewed published research. These are useful tools, but they cannot replace individual thought, experience, and imagination. I'm not suggesting you abandon your scientifically grounded internist, but that internist owes you, in exchange for your loyalty, a reasonable level of skepticism about mainstream dogma. If doctors, pressured by outside forces, buy into an approach saying exceptions to rules almost never happen, then they're liable to stop looking for those exceptions. If they don't look, we'll then face a self-fulfilling prophecy. If doctors say something doesn't happen, they'll never look for it and never see it happen. Even when it does, then they'll continue saying it doesn't happen with ever more conviction. When that happens, mainstream medical progress, the art and the science of it, will grind to a halt to the detriment of patient care.

Doctors and patients mired in the thyroid paradox can blame the misguided clinical simplism reviewed above, aided and abetted by an overly conservative academic elite of endocrinology. Leaders in the field have the knowledge to right many of the wrongs proposed in this book. I know they do because their publications support most of my points, yet they seem loath to bring what they know forward. Why? One reason could be the fear of error. They're terrified of doing harm. *Primum non nocere.* They refuse to advise any course unproven beyond an iota of doubt to be safe and effective. That reluctance—lack of clinical boldness, if you will— is born of both altruism and self-preservation. The positive motive to deliver only the best care possible and the selfish one to avoid punitive lawsuits when all does not go well.

Even when they personally believe in a course of action, and follow that course with their own patients, they hide behind evidence-based medicine when advising and teaching other physicians. Like the lecturer who said to me: "Rather than tell you my experience, let me tell you the literature." I recall another expert delivering a diatribe that boiled down to advice not to treat mild hypothyroidism with thyrotropin (TSH) levels that were only slightly greater than 5.0 mU/L. When pressed by an audience member, though, he jovially shrugged and said, "Well, I treat *everybody.*" Sure, tell me the evidence and let me judge for myself, but also tell me what you do in practice: if it's good enough for you and your patients, why not me and mine?

Besides the fear of error, there are other reasons the academic elite are slow to adopt—or at least advise—new ideas, tools, and methods. They are, for example, more disciplined scientists than typical community physicians, and they spend most of their days above the fray, teaching, writing, and administrating for their universities. When they see patients, it's often in the process of supervising medical students, residents, and fellows—a phalanx that puts in much of the actual face time with the patients, and that hears, for example, more of their bitter persisting complaints of fatigue and weight gain. Thus, many academic endocrinologists are relatively insulated from the intense experience of patient care. And it was that intense experience that taught me the lessons and fertilized the suspicions that led to *The Thyroid Paradox*. Am I a better or worse doctor for having begun to listen to my patients? Some of what I've written may turn out to be wrong, but I have to question whether the current leaders in the field are equipped to objectively make that judgment.

Patients want the straight scoop; in a sense, when they turn to an alternative medicine practitioner or order pills over the Internet in response to unproven claims of healthfulness, these patients are begging doctors not to be so stubbornly circumspect. I'm not suggesting that doctors should ignore their obligation to do the "right thing" just because some patients want them to. What I am saying is that, in medicine, as much harm can come from acting too late as too early. The patient who abandons her internist in favor of an alternative practitioner (an iridologist, for example, or someone offering ion foot baths) might have done so solely because she feels the internist has persistently ignored her concerns. Better listening, a few more tests, perhaps coloring just a little outside the lines of strict standard practice might have saved the therapeutic relationship between that internist and his or her patient. Dogmatism is the mutual worst enemy of that doctor and patient. Caution is warranted, but not to the point of clinical stagnation.

Hypothyroidism comes in many varieties. Most doctors, though, don't think beyond obvious primary hypothyroidism, which is an unquestionably commonplace condition. Despite how common it is, though, and despite this focus, doctors still miss many actual cases of primary hypothyroidism. The secret to uncovering most of those missed cases, I think, lies in simply changing the rules for interpreting thyroid blood tests. By and large, these tests work for primary hypothyroidism, provided they are read correctly.

But even if all those cases of typical hypothyroidism get picked up, that will still leave undiagnosed the atypical forms of low thyroid: mostly central hypothyroidism and thyroid hormone resistance. Central hypothyroidism, in particular, is probably a lot less rare than most doctors think. It's a condition that is very good at hiding from the usual blood tests, no matter how creatively doctors interpret them, and it might be triggered by such ubiquitous conditions as stress, depression, and obesity. Listening to the patient's history, regardless of the test numbers, may be the only way to ferret out these cases.

What can you as a low-thyroid patient, or a potential one, do to escape the thyroid paradox? Unfortunately, for most problems I've outlined in this book, there are no do-it-yourself diet changes, or exercises, or supplements that offer reliable fixes. And I strongly advise you not to start on, or make changes in dosages of, drugs like Synthroid without the personal supervision of a licensed healthcare provider. The solutions I espouse by and large require a doctor to make the right diagnosis, then prescribe the right dose(s) of the right medication(s)—and for the patient to take that medication as advised and report back any problems, benefits, or failures. In other words, the path out of the thyroid paradox is engaged teamwork involving both doctor and patient. This book should provide you with the knowledge you need to communicate and work with, and perhaps even educate, your doctor in order to get this teamwork ball rolling.

Obviously, for you, the first step is to find a doctor willing to be half of that team. That doctor may turn out to be the one you have now, or you may need to seek a second or third opinion. It may be a simple matter of asking your current doctor for a referral or you may have to do your own search. Ask friends or family with thyroid problems for recommendations. They may have been over the same ground you're treading. I can't tell you what kind of doctor would be your best partner; it depends too much on the individual. In general though, the more a doctor knows about thyroidology and the longer he or she has been in practice, the better. A very experienced endocrinologist often will fill that bill best. I'd probably avoid nurse practitioners, physician's assistants, and doctors who are less than five years (perhaps even ten years) out of training—these professionals may tend to be too married to evidence-based medicine and unwavering standards. I'd also steer clear of university settings. None of these, however, are hard and fast rules. Try calling a prospective new doctor's office and asking simple screening questions before committing to and waiting for an appointment: "Does he or she ever prescribe combined T_4/T_3 therapy?" or "Does he or she ever give thyroid pills in spite of normal lab results?" Don't word the question "*Will* he do so and so . . .?" No honest, competent physician would promise a certain treatment to a perfect stranger without first doing an evaluation.

If you're seeing your thyroid doctor for other things, by the way (as will often be the case if it's your internist or family practitioner that you're seeing about your thyroid), you might make a separate special appointment at least once just to talk about thyroid issues. The more time and focus the doctor can devote to one problem, the more listening and thinking outside the box you'll get for your trouble.

Assuming you're reasonably sure you're working with an open-minded doctor who is listening to your concerns, ask if the physician would consider a short trial of thyroid hormone just to see if it helps, or if you're on thyroid pills, ask to try out a higher dose even if the numbers are "normal." There is little risk of harm in giving average doses of levothyroxine for a few weeks to otherwise healthy adults, particularly young adults. Any doctor not stuck like glue to some clinical cookbook should realize this and be willing to try the intervention and monitor the outcome. If the physician refuses, ask why. Remember to try to be as flexible and open-minded as a patient as you're asking your doctor to be. He or she may have other suggestions—other conditions to test for or treatments to recommend. Ask about future plans—"What if this doesn't work, then what?"—and make bargains. "I'll take these extra tests, but if we don't find anything, I'd really like to try thyroid hormone. Okay?"

I recall a patient who came to me adamant that she wanted to take

Armour Thyroid—a product I don't usually prescribe. I explained why, discussed the pros and cons of various ways of giving thyroid replacement, and convinced her to just try a higher dose of Synthroid. I also promised to do it her way if my ideas didn't pan out. More Synthroid, in fact, did her no good. I added Cytomel, which didn't seem to help either, so eventually, as promised, I gave her Armour Thyroid. That worked. She's now a happy patient and I feel I did the right thing by trying more standard therapies before going to less standard ones. Open-mindedness, communication, and trust—on both our parts—made that relationship work.

CONCLUSION

The following are my recommendations and caveats regarding management of hypothyroidism. They are my opinions and should be afforded no more or less weight than the reader feels is warranted at this point.

- Top endocrinologists should impress upon specialists and primary-care providers alike the significance of the entire thyroid system, not just the hypothalamic-pituitary-thyroid (HPT) axis.

- They should also spotlight the weaknesses of modern thyroid blood testing outside the narrow scope of classic primary hypothyroidism.

- Normal test results do not equal normal patients.

- In hypothyroidism, clinical evaluation is just as critical as blood testing.

- Thyrotropin (TSH) levels greater than 2.0 mU/L aren't normal.

- Most mildly high TSH levels (greater than 5.0 mU/L), even if T_4 and T_3 tests are normal, should be treated, and treatment should be considered for TSH levels greater than 2.0 mU/L.

- In the early phases of any thyroid workup, both free thyroxine and TSH tests should be done. The relationship between the two might be the only clue to subtle problems.

- In a possibly hypothyroid patient, or one already on replacement therapy, when "normal" lab tests disagree with clinical findings, the possibility of a hidden abnormality in the thyroid system (for example, central hypothyroidism or thyroid hormone resistance) must be considered.

- Thought to be rare, central hypothyroidism might instead be common, but grossly underdiagnosed.

- Some central hypothyroidism might be caused by everyday stress, anxiety, or depression.

- Although resistance to thyroid hormone exists, it is almost never considered. It might be rare or it might be common, and some parts of the body can be more resistant than others, making symptoms and tests very difficult to decipher.

- In a patient on thyroid replacement therapy, an undetectably low TSH level usually means the thyroid hormone dose needs to be lowered, but not always.

- In a low-thyroid patient who has been treated in the past for high thyroid, TSH levels are often misleadingly low, leaving the thyroid's gas gauge stuck on "F" and leading to undertreatment.

- Full-replacement dosing might prevent some poor responses to thyroid replacement therapy.

- Another reason for failure of, or intolerance to, thyroid replacement therapy might be the unmasking of nonthyroid problems—including poor physical fitness, anxiety, and heart disease—by the correction of hypothyroidism. In other words, correction of one problem (low thyroid) might worsen or expose other problems that have to be dealt with separately.

- Some people on levothyroxine (LT$_4$)–only replacement therapy might benefit from adding liothyronine (LT$_3$).

- Thyroid failure isn't "the Big One," nor is it simple or inconsequential.

In correcting the thyroid paradox, and increasing their willingness to label and treat more obscure examples of hypothyroidism, doctors must guard against riding this pendulum too far in the other direction. Doctors too willing to reject normal lab tests may massively overtreat patients. At what peril? At the least, the risk of escalating healthcare costs. At the worst, well, if anything is worse than a serious side effect caused by a needed therapy, it's one triggered by an unneeded therapy.

In a scene from the film *Jurassic Park*, Jeff Goldblum's character berates the creator of a slew of cloned dinosaurs, arguing that just because something can be done doesn't mean it should be done. I offer the same caution about thyroid replacement therapy outside established standards of care: it can be done and in some cases should be, but only after careful consideration. Reckless prescribing cannot be supported.

Some low-thyroid patients are easy to spot and treat, just as main-streamists say. Some are hard to spot and treat, but can be detected when doctors use their diagnostic tools to maximum effect. Some patients are just plain invisible to those tools and require clinical cunning, just as reformists say. Have we resolved the thyroid paradox? Probably not. Nar-rowed the gulf between reformists and mainstreamists? I hope so. The truth is out there, somewhere in the middle.

If you're frustrated, believing you're stuck in the thyroid paradox, take heart. This book may arm you with the information and advice you need to find your way out. The key is, don't be satisfied with business-as-usual health care. Don't accept a clinical practice guideline or evidence-based medicine as the final arbiter of your diagnosis and treatment. Don't be sat-isfied with doctors who don't listen to your concerns or take the time to discuss them. Don't accept the answer "It's not your thyroid" on its face. Many of my patients who were originally told that now live symptom free, or at least improved, lives after starting new or modified thyroid therapy. Clearly, I can't promise that you will find your answer in these pages, but you might, and even an open-minded trial of thyroid therapy that fails is useful, because it will free you to explore other possibilities, using your now enhanced team approach to working with your doctor.

EPILOGUE

While I was working on *The Thyroid Paradox*, I attended the 2006 Endocrine Society meeting in Boston. Scientifically and clinically, the conference was outstanding. I learned a few new things—some of which will change my practice for the better—and got soothing reassurance that most of what I do is still considered correct.

As for the mainstream approach to the challenges of diagnosing and treating hypothyroidism, little has changed. Combination therapy using T_3 is still largely condemned. Treating TSH levels not exceeding 10.0 milliunits per liter (mU/L) is still controversial to varying degrees, depending on which expert is on stage talking at the moment. And with respect to the patient with thyroid-like complaints whose tests are "normal," the answer still is "It's not your thyroid."

I am very pleased to report, however, what I perceive to be a marked shift in attitude. The messages were the same, but they were more often couched in a compassionate recognition that the "thyroid paradox" patient is out there. There was acknowledgment that she deserves a fair hearing of her concerns, whether or not they are truly thyroid-related, and that doctors' dismissals of such concerns alienate people, possibly harmfully, away from mainstream medicine (a discipline that paradoxically professes, above all, "first, do no harm"); that, for example, a well-supervised trial of T_3 therapy might be safe, reasonable, and valuable to the patient and to the quality of her relationship with her doctor, even if that doctor is pretty sure it won't do her any good; and that doctors are—or should be—as much healers as they are scientists.

Alternative therapies as a whole, while not embraced, seemed to be viewed at this conference in a more practical light. Patients are taking them, whether mainstream doctors like it or not, and some may be helpful, some may be harmful, and some may be neither. Speakers made the point that doctors have a responsibility to understand those therapies and be open-minded. One lecturer admonished us to discuss an alternative therapy as either "proven" or "unproven," but not to automatically label it as worthless or dangerous just because it is not FDA-approved or available by standard prescription.

Finally, I was impressed by a plenary lecture (a session reserved for the most important presentations of general interest) attended by a few thousand endocrinologists and other physicians. The talk was on T_4/T_3 combination therapy, and I've already told you what it concluded. The speaker, however, closed by describing a formal complaint lodged with a member of the British Parliament and the United Kingdom's General Medical Council "against the clinical practice of the majority of the medical profession with regard to the diagnosis and management of hypothyroidism on four counts . . . ." As quoted in the British medical journal *Clinical Endocrinology*, those four counts were:

1. Over-reliance on thyroid blood tests and a total lack of reliance on signs, symptoms, history of the patient, and a clinical appraisal.

2. The emotional abuse and blatant disregard by the majority of general practitioners and endocrinologists over the suffering experienced by untreated/incorrectly treated thyroid patients and their lack of compassion over the fate of these patients.

3. Stubbornness of general practitioners and endocrinologists to treat patients suffering from hypothyroidism with a level of medication that returns the patient to optimum health. In addition, the unwillingness to prescribe alternate thyroid treatment for patients on individual grounds . . . such as Armour Thyroid.

4. The ongoing reluctance to encourage debate or further research on hypothyroidism.

Or, for brevity's sake, we could simply say that those four counts are, word for word, a condensed version of *The Thyroid Paradox*.

Hope springs eternal . . .

GLOSSARY

Adrenal glands. Two glands, one above each kidney, that produce steroids and epinephrine (adrenaline).

Antibodies. Proteins usually produced as a reaction to the body's exposure to a foreign particle; they flag the object for destruction by the immune system.

Armour Thyroid. Brand name of thyroid USP.

Autoantibodies. Antibodies that bind inappropriately to a part of one's own body; their presence may indicate the patient has an autoimmune disease.

Autoimmune. Adjective describing the state in which one's immune system inappropriately attacks some part of one's own body; many diseases are autoimmune in nature.

Biochemical evaluation. Blood tests.

Biochemical hypothyroidism. Low-thyroid state indicated by blood tests alone.

Central hypothyroidism. Low-thyroid state caused by poor or absent stimulation of the thyroid gland by the hypothalamic-pituitary-thyroid (HPT) axis; contrast with primary hypothyroidism.

Clinical exam. The hands-on portion of a medical evaluation—what the doctor sees, hears, or feels at the bedside or in the clinic; contrast with biochemical evaluation.

Clinical hypothyroidism. Low-thyroid state indicated by clinical findings alone or any collection of signs and symptoms that strongly suggest a low-thyroid state.

Clinical practice guideline. Document published by a medical organization defining and promoting the group's consensus opinion on the proper way to manage a certain health problem, such as hypothyroidism.

Corticotropin-releasing hormone. Hormone produced by the hypothalamus involved in regulation of the adrenal glands.

Cortisol. One of the major steroid hormones produced by the adrenal glands. *See* glucocorticoid.

CRH. *see* Corticotropin-releasing hormone.

Cushing's syndrome. Disease state caused by too much glucocorticoid in the blood.

Cytomel. Brand name of liothyronine (LT_3).

Deiodinase. Enzyme located in many organs throughout the body that activates or deactivates thyroid hormone depending on the needs of the moment.

Desiccated thyroid. Thyroid USP.

DNA. The biochemical substance that forms the genetic blueprints of life; most cells in the human body contain a complete copy of the individual's DNA organized into forty-six chromosomes.

Dyslipidemia. Abnormalities in cholesterol and/or triglyceride levels that can lead to heart disease and stroke.

Endocrine. Referring to the endocrine glands.

Endocrine gland. Organ that secretes a hormone directly into the blood.

Endocrinologist. An M.D. or D.O. specializing in endocrinology; endocrinologists who are board-certified (not all are) have completed a two- or three-year fellowship training program after internal medicine residency and passed a certifying exam given by the American Board of Internal Medicine.

Endocrinology. Subspecialty of internal medicine involving disorders of endocrine glands and certain bone diseases.

End-organ effect. Any hormone effect.

Enzyme. Any of a large number of proteins in the body that regulate chemical reactions.

False positive. A test result that is positive for a disease when the person tested does not actually have that disease.

Follicular cells. In the thyroid gland, epithelial cells that form the outer shell of the thyroid follicle; they produce and secrete thyroid hormone.

Free hormone hypothesis. The notion that only hormones loose in the blood, not bound to serum proteins, are available to bind to receptors and carry out their actions.

Generalist. A physician who is not a specialist; a primary-care provider (PCP).

Gland. Any organ that secretes something within or outside the body.

Glucocorticoid. Important class of steroid hormones that are necessary for life; blood levels increase during physical or emotional stress, especially severe injury or illness; controls blood pressure and sugar and fat metabolism; synthetic versions are often used as drugs.

Goiter. Any abnormally enlarged thyroid gland.

Hashimoto's thyroiditis. A chronic autoimmune thyroid disease often causing goiter and/or hypothyroidism; thought to be the most common cause of unexpected hypothyroidism; also called chronic autoimmune thyroiditis or chronic lymphocytic thyroiditis.

Hormone. Any chemical substance produced in one part of the body that is transported to another part via blood to exert some form of control.

Hormone effect. Intended result of a hormone's release and eventual binding to its receptor; for thyrotropin (TSH), the hormone effect is thyroid hormone release; thyroid hormone has numerous effects, for example, increased body heat production.

HPT axis. *See* Hypothalamic-pituitary-thyroid axis.

Hyperthyroidism. Too much thyroid hormone in the blood.

Hypothalamic-pituitary-thyroid (HPT) axis. One of the principal systems regulating thyroid hormone production; the hypothalamus makes TRH, stimulating the pituitary gland to make TSH, which stimulates the thyroid gland to make thyroid hormone; each product along the path blocks further production of its own stimulator.

Hypothalamus. Area at the center of the brain that regulates a number of basic body functions, including appetite and metabolism.

Hypothyroidism. Low-thyroid state.

Individual reference range. For a blood test, the span between the lowest and the highest numerical measurements when a test is run on the same person multiple times; it is typically narrower than the true reference range, which is determined using one test each run on many people, instead of many tests run on one person; it boils down to a statistical recognition that people are different—just because your result is normal for the population doesn't mean it's normal for you.

Iodine. Critical nutrient used by the body to produce thyroid hormone.

Levothroid. A brand name of levothyroxine.

Levothyroxine. Drug containing thyroxine (T_4) as its only active ingredient; manufactured under several brand names and as a generic drug.

Levoxyl. A brand name of levothyroxine.

Liothyronine. Drug containing triiodothyronine (T_3) as its only active ingredient; manufactured under the brand name Cytomel.

LT$_3$. *See* Liothyronine.

LT$_4$. *See* Levothyroxine.

Mainstreamist. For the purposes of this book, a doctor who manages thyroid patients in more-or-less strict accordance with current standards, published clinical practice guidelines and peer-reviewed research, and the teachings of top medical school professors; connotation can be good or bad—implies close-mindedness but also prudence in what the physician does for and to patients; contrast with reformist.

Myxedema. Old term for hypothyroidism; specifically refers to skin thickening typical of severe low-thyroid states.

NHANES III. Third National Health and Nutrition Examination Survey; a huge study managed by the U.S. Centers for Disease Control, conducted between 1988 and 1994, designed to estimate the health and nutritional status of the United States population across all ages.

Normal range. Often and somewhat incorrectly used to mean reference range; reference range is a statistical concept defining frequency in a group of people, but not necessarily "normal" health; for example, obesity is frequent, but not physiologically normal or healthy.

Nucleus. Structure inside most of the body's cells that houses their DNA.

PCP. *See* Primary-care provider.

Peripheral conversion. Chemical change of the prohormone T_4 into the active hormone T_3 in the liver, kidneys, brain, muscles, and other areas outside the thyroid gland; mediated by deiodinase; along with the HPT axis, one of the principal systems regulating thyroid hormone action.

PHCH. *See* Post-hyperthyroid central hypothyroidism.

Pituitary gland. Bulblike structure at the end of a stalk extending from the bottom of the hypothalamus; secretes numerous hormones, many of which regulate other endocrine glands, including the thyroid; often called the master gland.

Post-hyperthyroid central hypothyroidism. Central hypothyroidism caused by permanent or temporary HPT axis suppression by high thyroid hormone levels

Primary-care provider. Any doctor a patient sees for most routine medicine care, physical exams, and health maintenance; for adults, this role is usually filled by an internist or family practitioner.

Primary hypothyroidism. Low-thyroid state caused by destruction of or defect within the thyroid gland itself; contrast with central hypothyroidism.

Prohormone. Immature, less active, or inactive form of a hormone.

Radioactive iodine. Any radioactive isotope (form) of iodine; iodine-123, a low-energy isotope is used in nuclear medicine thyroid scanning; iodine-131, which has a higher, more destructive output, is often used in treatment of hyperthyroidism and thyroid cancer.

Receptor. The site of attachment of a hormone in or on its target cell; once the hormone binds to it, the receptor signals other structures to begin carrying out a preprogrammed set of events that result in the desired end-organ effect.

Reference range. For a blood test, the span of numerical results considered to be normal or at least most frequently obtained, as defined and published by the laboratory running the test; typically the middle 95 percent of results when the test is run on a group of healthy people. *See* normal range.

Reformist. For the purposes of this book, anyone—perhaps an M.D. but often not—who believes in and promotes management of true or perceived thyroid disease in a manner contrary to mainstreamist practice; the connotation can be good or bad: the term implies healthy open-mindedness about how to do things but also recklessness in patient care and rejection of the scientific method of inquiry.

RTH. *See* Thyroid hormone resistance.

Scientific method. A disciplined system of inquiry that begins with a hypothesis (a tentatively assumed truth), then proceeds to experimentation to test that hypothesis, the gathering of data from the experiment, and the interpretation of that data with respect to the actual truth or falsehood of the original hypothesis;

mainstreamists tend to require their beliefs to hold up to this standard, while reformists may not.

Sensitivity. For any test, the percentage of people with the disease in question who have a positive result—that is, positivity in disease.

Sign. Any clinical finding objectively observed by a doctor; for example, a coughing fit seen by the doctor is a sign; contrast with symptom.

Specificity. For any test, the percentage of people without the disease in question who have a negative result—that is, negativity in the absence of disease.

Steroid. Any member of a large family of chemical substances with the same cholesterol-based molecular backbone; many are hormones (such as cortisol, estrogen, testosterone, and vitamin D) and many are used as drugs, including the anabolic steroids used illegally by some athletes.

Symptom. Any clinical finding described by the patient to the doctor; "I had a coughing fit last night" would be a symptom; contrast with sign.

Synthroid. A brand name of levothyroxine; the first LT_4 marketed and currently the most widely prescribed.

T_3. *See* Triiodothyronine.

T_4. *See* Thyroxine.

Target cell. For any given hormone, any cell in the body that binds and responds to it.

TBG. *See* Thyroxine-binding globulin.

Thermogenesis. Internal body-heat production typical of mammals and birds; stimulated by thyroid hormone.

Thyroglobulin. Protein produced by thyroid follicular cells from which thyroid hormone is derived.

Thyroid antibodies. Autoantibodies directed against parts of the thyroid gland; their presence may indicate autoimmune thyroid disease.

Thyroid follicle. Self-contained unit within the thyroid gland responsible for the manufacture, storage, and secretion of thyroid hormone.

Thyroid function test. Any blood test used to determine if thyroid system function is normal.

Thyroid gland. Organ in the neck that manufactures, stores, and releases thyroid hormone into the blood.

Thyroid hormone. Hormone produced by the thyroid gland that has a key role in regulation of total body metabolism, nervous system function, and generation of body heat.

Thyroid hormone resistance. Low-thyroid state caused by a defect in the thyroid system (*see* below) after thyroid hormone secretion by the thyroid gland, resulting in tissue hypothyroidism but not biochemical hypothyroidism; typically the problem is genetic damage to the thyroid hormone receptor.

Thyroid nodule. Tumor of the thyroid gland; usually benign, but can be malignant.

Thyroidology. Scientific study of and medical focus on the thyroid system.

Thyroidologist. Any M.D. or D.O., but usually an endocrinologist, whose practice focuses on thyroid disease; an informal term, not an official subspecialty.

Thyroid paradox. The odd observation that hypothyroidism is a very common disease that is nonetheless greatly underdiagnosed.

Thyroid replacement therapy (TRT). Prescription drug treatment of a low-thyroid state, usually with levothyroxine or Thyroid USP.

Thyroid-stimulating hormone (TSH). Thyrotropin.

Thyroid system. Collection of organs and processes within the body involved in the generation of thyroid hormone and its end-organ effects; major components include the HPT axis, the thyroid gland, serum transport proteins such as TBG, and the target cells.

Thyroid USP. Drug containing T_4 and T_3 derived from the dried thyroid glands of animals.

Thyrotropin. Hormone produced by the pituitary gland that regulates thyroid gland production and release of thyroid hormone.

Thyrotropin-releasing hormone (TRH). Hormone produced by the hypothalamus that regulates pituitary gland production and release of thyrotropin.

Thyroxine (T_4). The more abundant, less potent major form of thyroid hormone in the blood; prohormone of T_3.

Thyroxine-binding globulin (TBG). One of the major thyroid hormone transport proteins.

Tissue hypothyroidism. Inadequate T_3 reaching the target cell; may or may not be accompanied by biochemical hypothyroidism (abnormal blood tests), but often causes clinical hypothyroidism (signs and symptoms).

Transport proteins. Proteins in the blood that bind thyroid hormone, forming a vast reserve of T_4 and T_3 spread throughout the body.

Treatment threshold. For any blood test, the level of abnormality required before therapy is started.

TRH. *See* Thyrotropin-releasing hormone.

TRH-stim test. *See* TRH-stimulation test.

TRH-stimulation test. A test, usually done in an endocrinologist's office, in which TRH is injected and the resulting rise in TSH, if any, is measured; the "gold standard" test for HPT axis function; as of this writing, not available routinely in the United States.

Triiodothyronine (T_3). The less abundant, more potent major form of thyroid hormone in the blood; mostly formed from thyroxine via peripheral conversion.

TRT. *See* Thyroid replacement therapy.

TSH. *See* Thyroid-stimulating hormone or thyrotropin.

Unithroid. A brand name of levothyroxine.

Zulewski list. A list of twelve common findings in low-thyroid patients; the presence of six or more of the items in a patient is highly suggestive of true hypothyroidism.

REFERENCES

Introduction

Hollowell, J., et al. "Serum TSH, T_4, and Thyroid Antibodies in the United States Population (1988 to 1994): National Health and Nutritional Examination Survey (NHANES III)." *Journal of Clinical Endocrinology and Metabolism* 87 (2002): 489–499.

Montori, V. "Evidence-based Endocrine Practice." *Endocrine Practice* 9 (2003): 321–323.

Naylor, C. "Grey Zones of Clinical Practice: Some Limits to Evidence-based Medicine." *Lancet* 345 (1995): 840–842.

Rizz, R., et al. "A Model to Determine Workforce Needs for Endocrinologists in the United States Until 2020." *Journal of Clinical Endocrinology and Metabolism* 88 (2003): 1979–1987.

Vanderpump, M., and W. Tunbridge. "The Epidemiology of Thyroid Diseases." In Braverman, L., and R. Utiger (eds.). *Werner and Ingbar's The Thyroid: A Fundamental and Clinical Text*, 8th ed. Philadelphia: Lippincott, Williams & Wilkins, 2000, pp. 467–473.

Chapter 1

Chopra, I., and L. Sabatino. "The Nature and Sources of Circulating Thyroid Hormones." In Braverman, L., and R. Utiger (eds.). *Werner and Ingbar's The Thyroid: A Fundamental and Clinical Text*, 8th ed. Philadelphia: Lippincott, Williams & Wilkins, 2000, pp. 121–131.

Chapter 2

Al-Adsani, H., L. Hoffer, and J. Silva. "Resting Energy Expenditure is Sensitive to

171

Small Dose Changes in Patients on Chronic Thyroid Hormone Replacement." *Journal of Clinical Endocrinology and Metabolism* 82 (1997): 1118–1125.

American Academy of Family Physicians. *Summary of Policy Recommendations for Periodic Health Examinations.* Reprint No. 510. Leawood, KS: American Academy of Family Physicians, 2002.

Helfand, M., C. Redfern, and H. Sox. "Screening for Thyroid Disease." *Annals of Internal Medicine* 129 (1998): 141–143.

Knudsen, N., et al. "Small Differences in Thyroid Function May Be Important for Body Mass Index and the Occurrence of Obesity in the Population." *Journal of Clinical Endocrinology and Metabolism* 90 (2005): 4019–4024.

Ladenson, P., et al. "American Thyroid Association Guidelines for Detection of Thyroid Dysfunction." *Archives of Internal Medicine* 160 (2000): 1708–1709.

U.S. Preventive Services Task Force. "Screening for Thyroid Disease: Recommendation Statement." *Annals of Internal Medicine* 140 (2004): 125–127.

Zulewski, et al. "Estimation of Tissue Hypothyroidism by a New Clinical Score: Evaluation of Patients with Various Grades of Hypothyroidism and Controls." *Journal of Clinical Endocrinology and Metabolism* 82 (1997): 771–777.

Chapter 3

Barnes, B., and L. Galton. *Hypothyroidism: The Unsuspected Illness.* New York: Harper & Row, 1976.

Baskin, H., et al. "American Association of Clinical Endocrinologists Medical Guidelines for Clinical Practice for the Evaluation and Treatment of Hyperthyroidism and Hypothyroidism." *Endocrine Practice* 8 (2002): 457–469.

Biondi, B., et al. "Effects of Subclinical Thyroid Dysfunction on the Heart." *Annals of Internal Medicine* 137 (2002): 904–914.

Demers, L., and C. Spencer. "Laboratory Medicine Practice Guidelines: Laboratory Support for the Diagnosis and Monitoring of Thyroid Disease." *Thyroid* 13 (2003): 3–126.

Helfand, M., C. Redfern, and H. Sox. "Screening for Thyroid Disease." *Annals of Internal Medicine* 129 (1998): 141–143.

Ross, D. "Subclinical Hypothyroidism." In Braverman, L., and R. Utiger (eds.). *Werner and Ingbar's The Thyroid: A Fundamental and Clinical Text,* 8th ed. Philadelphia: Lippincott, Williams & Wilkins, 2000, pp. 1001–1006.

Vanderpump, M., and W. Tunbridge. "Epidemiology and Prevention of Clinical and Subclinical Hypothyroidism." *Thyroid* 12 (2002): 839–847.

Chapter 4

Andersen, S., et al. "Narrow Individual Variations in Serum T_4 and T_3 in Normal Subjects: A Clue to the Understanding of Subclinical Thyroid Disease." *Journal of Clinical Endocrinology and Metabolism* 87 (2002): 1068–1072.

Demers, L., and C. Spencer. "Laboratory Medicine Practice Guidelines: Laboratory Support for the Diagnosis and Monitoring of Thyroid Disease." *Thyroid* 13 (2003): 3–126.

Dickey, R., L. Wartofsky, and S. Feld. "Optimal Thyrotropin Level: Normal Ranges and Reference Intervals are Not Equivalent." *Thyroid* 15 (2005): 1035–1039.

Hollowell, J., et al. "Serum TSH, T_4, and Thyroid Antibodies in the United States Population (1988 to 1994): National Health and Nutritional Examination Survey (NHANES III)." *Journal of Clinical Endocrinology and Metabolism* 87 (2002): 489–499.

Surks, M., G. Goswami, and G. Daniels. "The Thyrotropin Reference Range Should Remain Unchanged." *Journal of Clinical Endocrinology and Metabolism* 90 (2005): 5489–5496.

Vanderpump, M., et al. "The Incidence of Thyroid Disorders in the Community: A Twenty-year Follow-up of the Whickham Survey." *Clinical Endocrinology* 43 (1995): 55–68.

Vanderpump, M., and W. Tunbridge. "The Epidemiology of Thyroid Diseases." In Braverman, L., and R. Utiger (eds.). *Werner and Ingbar's The Thyroid: A Fundamental and Clinical Text*, 8th ed. Philadelphia: Lippincott, Williams & Wilkins, 2000, pp. 467–473.

Wartofsky, L., and R. Dickey. "The Evidence for a Narrower Thyrotropin Reference Range is Compelling." *Journal of Clinical Endocrinology and Metabolism* 90 (2005): 5483–5488.

Chapter 5

Dluhy, R. "The Adrenal Cortex in Hypothyroidism." In Braverman, L., and R. Utiger (eds.). *Werner and Ingbar's The Thyroid: A Fundamental and Clinical Text*, 8th ed. Philadelphia: Lippincott, Williams & Wilkins, 2000, pp. 813–819.

Dluhy, R. "The Adrenal Cortex in Thyrotoxicosis." In Braverman, L., and R. Utiger (eds.). *Werner and Ingbar's The Thyroid: A Fundamental and Clinical Text*, 8th ed. Philadelphia: Lippincott, Williams & Wilkins, 2000, pp. 637–641.

Douyan, L., and D. Schteingart. "Effect of Obesity and Starvation on Thyroid

Hormone, Growth Hormone, and Cortisol Secretion." *Endocrinology and Metabolism Clinics of North America* 31 (2002): 173–189.

Habib, K., et al. "Neuroendocrinology of Stress." *Endocrinology and Metabolism Clinics of North America* 30 (2001): 695–728.

Martino, E., L. Bartalena, and A. Pinchera. "Central Hypothyroidism." In Braverman, L., and R. Utiger (eds.). *Werner and Ingbar's The Thyroid: A Fundamental and Clinical Text*, 8th ed. Philadelphia: Lippincott, Williams & Wilkins, 2000, pp. 762–773.

Tran, H. "Difficulties in Diagnosing and Managing Coexisting Primary Hypothyroidism and Resistance to Thyroid Hormone." *Endocrine Practice* 12 (2006): 288–293.

Chapter 6

Bartalena, L., and J. Robbins. "Variations in Thyroid Hormone Transport Proteins and Their Clinical Implications." *Thyroid* 2 (1992): 237–245.

Hollowell, J., et al. "Serum TSH, T_4, and Thyroid Antibodies in the United States Population (1988 to 1994): National Health and Nutritional Examination Survey (NHANES III)." *Journal of Clinical Endocrinology and Metabolism* 87 (2002): 489–499.

Köhrle, J., et al. "Selenium, the Thyroid, and the Endocrine System." *Endocrine Reviews* 26 (2005): 944–984.

Moriyama, K., et al. "Thyroid Hormone Action is Disrupted by Bisphenol A as an Antagonist." *Journal of Clinical Endocrinology and Metabolism* 87 (2002): 5185–5190.

Pardridge, W. "Transport of Thyroid Hormones into Tissues *in vivo*." In Wu, S. (ed.). *Current Issues in Endocrinology and Metabolism: Thyroid Hormone Metabolism—Regulation and Clinical Implications*. Boston: Blackwell Scientific Publications, 1991, pp. 123–143.

Refetoff, S. "Resistance to Thyroid Hormone." In Braverman, L., and R. Utiger (eds.). *Werner and Ingbar's The Thyroid: A Fundamental and Clinical Text*, 8th ed. Philadelphia: Lippincott, Williams & Wilkins, 2000, pp. 1028–1043.

Robbins, J. "Thyroid Hormone Transport Proteins and the Physiology of Hormone Binding." In Braverman, L., and R. Utiger (eds.). *Werner and Ingbar's The Thyroid: A Fundamental and Clinical Text*, 8th ed. Philadelphia: Lippincott, Williams & Wilkins, 2000, pp. 105–120.

Chapter 7

Al-Adsani, H., L. Hoffer, and J. Silva. "Resting Energy Expenditure is Sensitive to

Small Dose Changes in Patients on Chronic Thyroid Hormone Replacement." *Journal of Clinical Endocrinology and Metabolism* 82 (1997): 1118–1125.

Baran, D. "The Skeletal System in Thyrotoxicosis." In Braverman, L., and R. Utiger (eds.). *Werner and Ingbar's The Thyroid: A Fundamental and Clinical Text,* 8th ed. Philadelphia: Lippincott, Williams & Wilkins, 2000, pp. 659–666.

Bunevicius, R., et al. "Effects of Thyroxine as Compared with Thyroxine Plus Tri-iodothyronine in Patients with Hypothyroidism." *New England Journal of Medicine* 340 (1999): 424–429.

Greenspan, S., and F. Greenspan. "The Effect of Thyroid Hormone on Skeletal Integrity." *Annals of Internal Medicine* 130 (1999): 750–758.

Kaplan, M., D. Sarne, and A. Schneider. "Editorial: In Search of the Impossible Dream? Thyroid Hormone Replacement Therapy that Treats All Symptoms in All Hypothyroid Patients." *Journal of Clinical Endocrinology and Metabolism* 88 (2003): 4540–4542.

Keating, F., et al. "Treatment of Heart Disease Associated with Myxedema." *Progress in Cardiovascular Disease* 3 (1961): 364–381.

Rone, J., R. Dons, and H. Reed. "The Effect of Endurance Training on Serum Triiodothyronine Kinetics in Man: Physical Conditioning Marked by Enhanced Thyroid Hormone Metabolism." *Clinical Endocrinology* 37 (1992): 325–330.

Saravanan, P., et al. "Psychological Well-being in Patients on 'Adequate' Doses of L-thyroxine: Results of a Large, Community-based Questionnaire Study." *Clinical Endocrinology* 57 (2002): 577–585.

Sawka, A., et al. "Does a Combination Regimen of Thyroxine (T_4) and 3,5,3'-Tri-iodothyronine Improve Depressive Symptoms Better than T_4 Alone in Patients with Hypothyroidism? Results of a Double-blind, Randomized, Controlled Trial." *Journal of Clinical Endocrinology and Metabolism* 88 (2003): 4551–4555.

Singer, P., et al. "Treatment Guidelines for Patients with Hyperthyroidism and Hypothyroidism." *Journal of the American Medical Association* 273 (1995): 808–812.

Utiger, R. "Commentary on: Despite Adequate Thyroxine Therapy, Patients with Hypothyroidism Feel Less Well than Other Patients." *Clinical Thyroidology* 15 (2002): 8.

Walsh, J., et al. "Combined Thyroxine/Liothyronine Treatment Does Not Improve Well-being, Quality of Life, or Cognitive Function Compared to Thyroxine Alone: A Randomized Controlled Trial in Patients with Primary Hypothyroidism." *Journal of Clinical Endocrinology and Metabolism* 88 (2003): 4543–4550.

Chapter 8

Baskin, H., et al. "American Association of Clinical Endocrinologists Medical Guidelines for Clinical Practice for the Evaluation and Treatment of Hyperthyroidism and Hypothyroidism." *Endocrine Practice* 8 (2002): 457–469.

Cooper, D. "Combined T_4 and T_3 Therapy—Back to the Drawing Board." [Editorial] *Journal of the American Medical Association* 290 (2003): 3002–3004.

Kaplan, M., D. Sarne, and A. Schneider. "Editorial: In Search of the Impossible Dream? Thyroid Hormone Replacement Therapy that Treats All Symptoms in All Hypothyroid Patients." *Journal of Clinical Endocrinology and Metabolism* 88 (2003): 4540–4542.

Prummel, M., L. Brokken, and W. Wiersinga. "Ultra Short-loop Feedback Control of Thyrotropin Secretion." *Thyroid* 14 (2004): 825–828.

Sawin, C., et al. "Low Serum Thyrotropin Levels as a Risk Factor for Atrial Fibrillation in Older Persons." *New England Journal of Medicine* 331 (1994): 1249–1252.

Shimon, I., et al. "Thyrotropin Suppression by Thyroid Hormone Replacement is Correlated with Thyroxine Level Normalization in Central Hypothyroidism." *Thyroid* 12 (2002): 823–827.

Chapter 9

Hollowell, J., et al. "Serum TSH, T_4, and Thyroid Antibodies in the United States Population (1988 to 1994): National Health and Nutritional Examination Survey (NHANES III)." *Journal of Clinical Endocrinology and Metabolism* 87 (2002): 489–499.

Montori, V. "Evidence-based Endocrine Practice." *Endocrine Practice* 9 (2003): 321–323.

U.S. Preventive Services Task Force. "Screening for Thyroid Disease: Recommendation Statement." *Annals of Internal Medicine* 140 (2004): 125–127.

Epilogue

Weetman, A. "Whose Thyroid Replacement Is It Anyway?" *Clinical Endocrinology* 64 (2006): 231–233.

INDEX

ABOUT THE AUTHOR

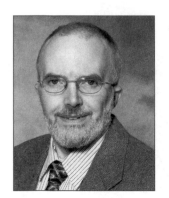

James K. Rone, M.D., is a writer and private-practice endocrinologist in Murfreesboro, Tennessee. He is a former military physician and has been awarded fellowship in both the American College of Physicians and the American College of Endocrinology. Thyroid disease—in particular hypothyroidism—has been his focus of clinical interest for nearly twenty years, and he is a thyroid patient himself, giving him a unique empathy for those struggling with thyroid disorders. He lives with his wife Susan on their farm outside Nashville.